Other titles by the authors:

The Nanny Connection: How to Find
and Keep the Perfect Nanny
by O. Robin Sweet

Sharing the Caring: How to Find the Right Child Care
and Make It Work for You
by Amy Laura Dombrow and Patty Bryan

The
Working
Woman's
Lamaze
Handbook

The Working Woman's Lamaze Handbook

The Essential Guide to Pregnancy, Lamaze, and Childbirth

by O. Robin Sweet and Patty Bryan

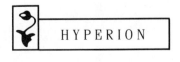

HYPERION

NEW YORK

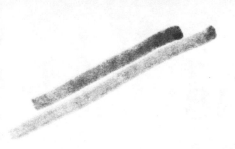

Library of Congress Cataloging-in-Publication Data

Sweet, O. Robin.
    The working woman's Lamaze handbook: the essential guide to pregnancy, Lamaze, and childbirth / by O. Robin Sweet and Patty Bryan.—1st ed.
        p.   cm.

ISBN 1-56282-976-9: $9.95 ($11.95 Can.)

1. Natural childbirth.   2. Pregnancy.   3. Pregnant women–Employment—United States.   I. Bryan, Patty.   II. Title.
RG661.S94   1992   92–3543
618.2'4—dc20   CIP

FIRST EDITION
10   9   8   7   6   5   4   3   2   1

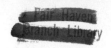
Dedication

I would like to dedicate this book to my husband, Thomas, who is the most incredibly supportive partner, and without whom my life would be incomplete.

I would also like to dedicate this book to my two beautiful daughters, Gretchen and Alexis, who are my constant source of inspiration.

A special dedication to my mother, Ottilie, who taught me the gentle art of mothering. Also, to both my parents, who instilled in me the theory that you can do anything that you set your mind to.

A final dedication to women everywhere who are contemplating having a family or who are pregnant at this time. We wish you much love and luck through the miraculous journey of pregnancy and childbirth.

O. Robin Sweet

Acknowledgments

Special thanks to:

Mike for all of his help. Dr. Beth Matlock, Gynecology, Infertility and Obstetrics Medical Group, Berkeley, California, for her instrumental medical editing. Carolyn Bass, OB/GYN head nurse at Windham Memorial Hospital. Maggie Halliday, R.N. and Lamaze instructor, Alta Bates-Herrick Hospital, Berkeley, California, for opening up her classroom and for her generosity and time. Stephanie Roteck for her beautiful illustrations. Sandra Jamroj, a Certified Childbirth Educator, Registered Movement Therapist, and teacher of Body-Mind-Centering (TM) and Terry Montemarno. Joe Spieler and Lisa Ross, our agents, for believing in our work. Leslie Wells (senior editor) and Ellen Cowhey (assistant) for their time and energy invested in making this work a success.

We would also like to thank the staff and public-relations department at Alta Bates-Herrick Hospital in Berkeley, California; Full Circle Childbirth and Midwifery Associates Perryn Reis and Ann Fuller; California Department of Health Services; American Academy of Pediatrics (California District); Peggy Vincent, Lamaze instructor; Marilyn Labrisco, Kaiser Hospital, Oakland, California; National Association of Childbirth Education; International Childbirth Education Association; Nurses Association of the American College of Obstetrics and Gynecology; James F. Erickson, EBD Group Associates, for the crucial insurance information; Johanna Peterson from the California Division of Occupational Safety and Health for her outstanding ability to produce information overnight; Employment Development Department; Dr. Barton Schmitt, National Parenting Center; and Terri Berthier, midwife.

Acknowledgments

We would also like to thank the many families that took the time to share their work, pregnancy, and childbirth experiences with us:

Bertie and David Alvarez, Lisa Evans and Derrick Clark, Don and Carol Steedman, Lynn Duncan and Robert Hrubes, Rob and Margaret McCall, Fred Diorazio and Evan Young, Beth and Robin Eiseman, Farshid and Taraneh Raafat, Sarah and Joseph Hamersky, Denise and Chris Pinto, Jon Raskin and Lori Lorenzo, Joy Fauvre and Greg Coplans, Antoinette Lavern, Lauren Clark, Angie Brown, Carol Einarsson, Connie Ashford, Kimberly Werner, Linda Clarke, Cheryl Coppola, Mary Laws, Sheila Cain, Roxie Chandler, Kelly Wilson, Dorothy Melendy, Kim Roman, Maryann Marshall, Kelly Wilson, Jay Lawrence, Joellyn Clark, Cynthia Robinson, K. Zuccarello, John Graham, Ranjan Sadarangani, A. Meisenheimer, Kathleen Nelson, Ann Toureilles, Janet Francom, Stephanie Beyer, Lesta Hall, Mary Ann Maclean, Kim Francis, R. Duncan, Cindy Bates, George Miklich, Brenda Withers, Sasha Goldberg, Jill Margolis, Sharon Collins, Heidi Beck, Denise Rusho, Nancy Armisto, Beth Sorenson, Jennifer Honaker, Lillie Downs, Pamela Haston, Samantha Jannke, and Cheryl Brown. If we have left anyone out, it was not intentional, and your information was truly valuable to the compilation of this book.

O. Robin Sweet and Patty Bryan

Contents

Contents

Contents

CHAPTER SEVEN: **Common Questions**
Questions 196

The
Working
Woman's
Lamaze
Handbook

INTRODUCTION

Most pregnant women are now working women as well. By the end of this century, half of the labor force in the United States will be female, and 85 percent of these women will become pregnant at some point in their working lives. *The Working Woman's Lamaze Handbook* is written for these prospective mothers. It is the only childbirth book to present the updated Lamaze method, everything else you need to know about pregnancy and childbirth, a complete exercise program, *and* also to address the specific concerns of working women—in one volume.

Most women want to take Lamaze classes. But one of the main complaints and concerns of pregnant working women is that they do not have time to attend the classes; trying to fit them into their busy schedules only adds stress to their lives. In addition, a coach is an integral part of the Lamaze method, and he or she needs to attend the classes too. That's a second busy schedule that has to be coordinated.

Lack of time and the difficulty of coordinating schedules are not the only factors that prevent working women from taking or completing childbirth classes. A secretary we know is typical. She had a toddler who was in child care all day. She felt guilty leaving her child with yet another sitter while she attended class, especially since the child was anxious about the upcoming new arrival. She also had to *find* that other sitter, which more often than not proved to be difficult and time-consuming. The classes and the sitter were a financial strain as well. And finally, like so many working women, pregnant or otherwise, she was so tired after a day on the job that going out again to do anything was a Herculean task. Who would want to take any course under these conditions? This woman somehow worked everything out and made all six evenings, but many do not. In fact, 50 percent of all Lamaze enrollees miss at least one class.

Perhaps you are in a similar situation. *The Working Woman's Lamaze Handbook* will make it possible for you to take your childbirth-preparation classes at any time or in any place that is convenient for you. You can read this book at home, on a lunch break, or relaxing in the tub. You will be provided with all of the information presented in your formal Lamaze courses, but you'll also be able to guide yourself and your coach through your own specialized course, as your schedules allow. The book can serve as a supplemental guide when you take a Lamaze course, but miss a class or two and have no way to make them up, and as a companion text if you simply want an easy-to-read companion guide for your classroom course.

The Lamaze method is relatively simple, whether presented in a class or in a book. This guide includes all of the basic Lamaze techniques that have been proven to help hundreds of thousands of women through labor and delivery. We divide the Lamaze material among the first six chapters so you can progress just as if you were attending the traditional six lessons of formal Lamaze courses. And if you use this book as a supplement to a classroom course, you will have no difficulty moving from classroom to book and back again. We *do* recommend that you take a class.

Lamaze courses have evolved so that most now provide much more than the basic breathing techniques. The information provided ranges from how to preregister at the hospital to how to interview a pediatrician; from what to take to the hospital to what to wear home; from what to use on stretch marks to the best kind of breast pump; from what kind of shoes to wear to how to fit exercises into one's daily schedule: hundreds of useful pieces of information. Lamaze classes now serve as clearinghouses for *any* kind of information relating to childbirth. *The Working Woman's Lamaze Handbook* will serve as such a resource, too.

As promised by the title, we will focus throughout the book on the unique needs of working women. Most working women are concerned about the security of their jobs. They worry about telling their bosses they are pregnant. They worry about discussing maternity leave, agreeing on a return date, whether they'll have the same job when they return, and whether they'll feel "out of sync." They worry about money and child care. Each chapter of this book devotes a section to these special concerns, and others, of working women. To provide indirect peer support, we include stories, anecdotes, and tips that helped women through job stress, as well as through pregnancy, labor, and delivery.

Introduction

The book is written to be appropriate whether your delivery will be in the hands of a physician or a midwife, but for simplicity's sake we will refer to the generic "doctor." The Lamaze breathing techniques call for the continuous presence during delivery of a husband, friend, midwife, relative, or doula. For simplicity's sake, again, we'll use the generic "coach" to designate this invaluable companion.

One important note: Lamaze classes usually begin between the thirtieth and thirty-fifth week. However, some of the problems and issues of pregnancy, especially those facing working women, begin much earlier than that. A good exercise program needs to be followed from the beginning. Therefore, most of the information we present in this book will be more beneficial if it is read and considered *early* in pregnancy—in the twelfth week, not the thirty-fifth. We recommend the book be read as soon as possible after pregnancy is established.

Each chapter is clearly divided into appropriate sections: Lamaze, Taking Care of Yourself, Work Issues, Exercises, and others as called for. Every chapter concludes with a list of recommended reading on pertinent subjects. In your initial first reading, you might skim the Lamaze sections and focus on the other material. Then, when the thirty-fifth week arrives, you'll be well prepared for focused work on the Lamaze technique. Those sections can be easily located in each chapter, one lesson per week. The other material in that chapter you will have absorbed and will be using already. We believe that the conscientious use of the information in this one book, on its own or in conjunction with Lamaze classes, will thoroughly prepare you and your coach for childbirth.

Class 1–Week 35

What's in This Chapter

Inside Info: Bladders, Bowels, and Breasts

Just Relax!

It Started in Russia

Lamaze Breathing: Slow-paced

Work Issues: Know Your Rights–The Pregnancy Discrimination Act

Taking Care of Yourself: No Time for Couch Potatoes

Inside Info: Bladders, Bowels, and Breasts

All about your innards: What a fun way to start a book! Unusual, too. But the inescapable first fact of pregnancy is that your body is going through astonishing changes. Whether you are ten weeks or thirty weeks pregnant, these changes are uppermost in your mind right now. They *are* pregnancy. At no other time in your life—or in anyone else's—is there an equivalent transformation. That is not too strong a word. Some of these changes you already know about because they're literally a pain—in the groin, for instance, or in your lower back. You will have to urinate more often than is convenient. You may well be constipated. Other changes mainly affect your emotions—those notorious hormones. And still other changes are so "internal" you might not notice them at all—in your cervix, for example—but they're important and you should understand them.

So let's cut straight to the chase in this first section: a part-by-part, hormone-by-hormone, complaint-by-complaint explanation of those miraculous changes going on in your body as you read these very words. Maybe the knowledge that your discomfort is all for a good cause will make you feel a little better.

Bladder: You have to urinate more often than you would like because your enlarging uterus is pressing on your bladder. In your last month, as the fetus reaches maximum size, you will feel even more pressure, and the urge to urinate will be even more pronounced (if you can believe it!).

Bowels: Your bowels are also being squeezed upward and backward by the growing fetus. This sounds awful, and it can indeed have an uncomfortable result: constipation. Exercise and a balanced diet are good preventives. However, if you are troubled by constipation, ask your doctor to prescribe appropriate medication.

Breasts: Your breasts seem to get bigger every day, and they ache all the time. They change constantly throughout your pregnancy, but once you deliver and your milk comes in, they go up yet another cup size. After delivery, they will be extra-sensitive. By wearing a bra that fits well, you can reduce the pulling and stretching on your chest and shoulders.

Breathing: As your pregnancy progresses, you will notice that you have more difficulty breathing. Again, this change is due to the enlarging fetus pushing up against your diaphragm. During the day, try to stand or sit in an upright position (not hunched over). This good posture (recommended at any time, for that matter) will give your lungs more room in which to expand, and the baby more room in which to move. Also, do some of the arm exercises found throughout this book. These create more room for the diaphragm. In bed, you can relieve some of your breathing problems by placing a couple of pillows under your head and shoulders so that you are almost in a sitting position. This position also gives your diaphragm a bit more room. If you can't sleep on your side, this is a great alternative.

Cervix: Your cervix probably isn't causing you any discomfort, but it plays an important role in your pregnancy. It's located in the lower segment of the uterus and looks like the bottom segment of a light bulb. As you get closer to your due date your cervix will begin effacing—the medical term for thinning out—and dilating, or opening up. These processes are necessary for your child to be born.

Digestion: As your pregnancy progresses, you will probably be disposed to heartburn, and your interest in eating might decline. Both conditions are caused by the growing fetus pushing your stomach up in your abdomen, where there isn't anywhere for it to go. So the stomach is squeezed. Avoiding fatty and spicy foods will help with the heartburn. There's really nothing to recommend for your loss of appetite, but it is important that you eat. Instead of eating a standard-sized meal three times a day, try eating six times a day and in smaller quantities.

Edema: Swelling of the legs is normal for most pregnant women. Edema is caused by fluid retention and by pressure from the uterus on the vena cava, a major vein returning blood from the legs to the heart. Thus your blood backs up in all the veins of the legs. Edema is not really of much concern *unless* accompanied by sudden puffiness or swelling of the hands, feet, or face. These can be signs of preeclampsia (see page 10). If this occurs, contact your doctor immediately.

Hemorrhoids: Occasionally pregnant women suffer from hemorrhoids, which are caused by the strain of carrying extra weight during pregnancy. These are varicose veins in the colon and rectum. They usually shrink and disappear after birth, but if you develop hemorrhoids, check with your doctor about taking a gentle stool softener.

Hormones: One minute you are very happy, and the next minute someone in your office says something that shouldn't bother you, but in fact causes you to burst into tears. Blame this on your hormones. Your body feels full and bloated, and your breasts have ached since your first month of pregnancy; hormones again. The levels of some of your regular hormones are increasing wildly, while new hormones are being produced by your body just for this pregnancy. For example, your progesterone level becomes ten times as high as before conception. In a single day, you produce as much estrogen as a nonpregnant woman produces in three years. According to one prominent textbook, *Williams Obstetrics,* during the course of a normal pregnancy you will produce as much estrogen as a nonpregnant woman would in 150 years! It's no wonder you're laughing one moment and crying the next.

Of course, these hormones have vital functions above just making pregnant women act in strange ways. Here are the major hormones and how they affect your pregnancy.

Estrogen: This essential female hormone promotes the growth of reproductive tissues by increasing the size of the uterus and the uterine lining, and by increasing the volume of blood and vaginal mucus. The high levels associated with pregnancy cause changes in breasts, uterus, vagina, metabolism (mainly the ability to break down sugars and carbohydrates), salt and water balance (water retention), and insulin secretion.

Human chorionic gonadotropin (HCG): This is one of the first hormones manufactured during pregnancy. It is thought to keep the mother's body from rejecting the embryo as foreign tissue, and to assure that the ovaries produce enough estrogen and progesterone until the placenta matures and assumes production of these hormones. It also causes boys' testes to produce the male hormone testosterone.

Placental lactogen (HPL): This hormone alters a mother's metabolism in order to make sugars and proteins more available to the growing fetus. It is believed to be the main hormone involved in the baby's growth. It also stimulates the areola (the dark part around the nipple) of the breasts in order to develop and prepare for lactation.

Progesterone: High levels of progesterone cause changes in the breasts, uterus, and vagina, and are thought to maintain pregnancy in the early phases and then to inhibit the frequency of uterine contractions during labor. Progesterone raises your body temperature and slows down your bowel, stomach, and bladder contractions. It also stimulates the secretion of the ovarian hormone relaxin.

Relaxin: This appropriately named hormone does what it says. It relaxes and softens the ligaments, cartilage, and cervix, allowing these tissues to spread during birth.

Epinephrine (adrenaline) and norepinephrine (noradrenaline) are commonly referred to as the "stress hormones." Anyone who's tense or excited produces them, and this definitely includes women in labor. They can affect the fetus by decreasing the blood flow to the mother's uterus and placenta, and they can prolong labor by decreasing the efficiency of uterine contractions. Relaxation and avoidance of caffeine are the best ways to prevent an oversupply of these hormones.

Linea Negra: You may notice a dark line running from your pubic area to your belly button. This line is called the *linea negra* and is thought to be caused by separation of your abdominal muscles. This is nothing to worry about, and disappears after the birth.

Lower Back: Your lower back will tend to ache, because of the tremendous pressure of the fetus on your sacrum and coccyx, and the added weight that your lower back is supporting. Pelvic-tilt exercises are marvelous for relieving this pressure and ache (see page 117). If you tuck a pillow under the largest part of your stomach and sleep on your side, you'll experience fewer backaches. Sleeping on your side during pregnancy is recommended by all doctors.

Pelvic-Floor Muscles: The pelvic-floor muscles are the hammock that supports your abdominal and pelvic organs. These muscles may sag due to the increased weight of your uterus and the relaxing effect of the hormones. Exercising them every day can maintain the tone of these muscles (see page 115).

Placenta: The placenta is flat and round, six to eight inches in diameter, according to the size of the baby. It weighs about one-seventh of the fetus's weight in a full-term delivery—roughly, one pound. Early in pregnancy it is the main source of estrogen and progesterone, but by the thirty-sixth week this hormone production decreases as the body prepares for the birth of the baby.

Preeclampsia: You may know of this condition as *toxemia* or, as it is currently sometimes called, *gestational edema-proteinuria-hypertension complex.* The terms are interchangeable. Preeclampsia occurs in about 5 to 10 percent of pregnancies, and usually in the latter half of pregnancy. It is more common in first-time mothers, and with women who have chronic diabetes, high blood pressure, or poor nutrition, or who are carrying twins. Preeclampsia is defined by a sudden and excessive fluid retention, rapid weight gain, high blood pressure, and protein in the urine. Some of the symptoms include headaches, visual problems, dizziness, or swelling of the ankles, face, or hands. If you have any of these symptoms, please contact your doctor.

Round Ligaments: Two round ligaments connect the front sides of the uterus to either side of the groin. The more you do the exercises for stretching and strengthening these ligaments, the easier your pregnancy and delivery will be. In fact, all the ligaments and cartilage of the pelvis must relax during pregnancy to allow greater mobility in the joints and to allow the pelvic bones to spread during labor and birth, giving your baby more room in the birth canal.

Have you had a sudden pain in the groin area when you made a sudden move or strained yourself by sneezing or coughing? This pain is probably caused by the sudden stretching of one or both of the round ligaments. You can help avoid these pains by moving slowly and, if you feel a sneeze coming on, by bending your knees and flexing your hips to relieve the strain.

Stretch Marks: Stretch marks are deep red marks that develop on your stomach, hips, or breasts during pregnancy, caused by the stretching of your skin. They will not remain dark red but will fade to a silver gray. Some women get the dark red marks, others only have tiny marks, and some women have no marks at all.

Varicose Veins: The pressure of the enlarging uterus impairs the return flow of venous blood from the legs, thus relaxing the walls of the blood vessels and creating varicose veins.

Uterus: Your uterus is making some radical changes during your pregnancy. The normal size of a uterus is two and a half inches long, one and a half inches wide, and one inch deep. At full term, your uterus is twelve and a half inches long, nine and a half inches wide, and eight and three-quarters inches deep. That's radical! It's also responsible for several of the complaints discussed in this section.

Weight Gain: The normal recommended weight gain during pregnancy is 25 to 35 pounds. Here's where those pounds and ounces are distributed:

Breasts: 0.9 pounds

Maternal blood: 2.8 pounds

Placenta: 1.4 pounds

Amniotic fluid: 1.8 pounds

Fetus: 7.7 pounds

Uterus: 2 pounds

Interstitial fluid: 2.7 pounds

Maternal tissue stores: 7.4 pounds

This hypothetical "itemization" totals 26.7 pounds. No single number is appropriate for every pregnant woman. If you were underweight before becoming pregnant, your doctor may encourage gaining extra weight. The latest statistics show that a greater weight

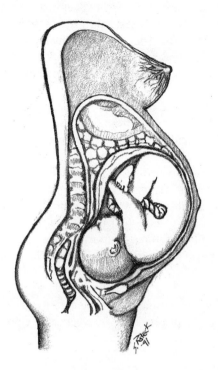

Ninth Month

gain during pregnancy results in more full-term pregnancies and larger, healthier babies. The issue of weight gain can be a touchy one; the main point to keep in mind is the importance of a healthy, well-balanced diet, to be discussed later in this chapter. If this diet is followed, the issue of how much weight to gain will just about take care of itself.

Just Relax!

The two most important principles of childbirth preparation presented in this book are the Lamaze breathing techniques and relaxation. From its very beginning, the Lamaze method assumed a relaxed body and a relaxed frame of mind as implied parts of the method. In recent years the trend has been toward more *explicit* instruction in some sort of relaxation technique. We agree. In fact, we feel so strongly about the importance of relaxation as a condition for effective Lamaze work that we introduce the subject now, prior to our introduction of Lamaze proper. Relaxation should not be a footnote in your preparation for childbirth; it should be a basic, ongoing program.

Just because someone tells you to relax doesn't necessarily mean that your body will respond. In fact, this instruction is more likely to make you tense because you have no earthly idea how to proceed. The ability to relax requires more than just telling your body to do it. Relaxation sounds simple enough, but when you're enduring the stresses of pregnancy, work, and childbirth, there's more to it than you think. It's a skill that must be learned.

Fortunately, relaxation techniques abound. Most YMCAs and YWCAs and health clubs offer courses in stress management or relaxation. Some corporations even have relaxation courses for their employees. Perhaps you have taken such a class and already know how beneficial some of these techniques can be. Doing an effective relaxation exercise can make you feel like a new person in as little as ten minutes.

If you're pregnant, it's *especially* important to find those ten minutes. And for working women, this can be especially difficult. Our friend Denise, an outside sales representative, found that the most convenient time for her to practice her relaxation techniques was driving to work. Obviously, she didn't close her eyes, and just as obviously, driving in a car isn't the best of all possible times, but it was the best Denise could do on many days, and it helped.

Can you be too tired to relax? Some women try to use that as an excuse, but we don't buy it. If nothing else, you can follow the practice of another friend, Sarah, who employed her relaxation images right before she went to sleep. We can understand how women may get uptight trying to figure out how to fit one more thing into their day's agenda, even something as pleasant as relaxation. But once they get into the habit, they're hooked. It makes the whole day easier.

Relaxation exercises during pregnancy serve a twofold purpose:

they will help you manage stress throughout your pregnancy, and they will serve as good practice for labor and delivery. You will need to release unnecessary tension between labor contractions. Relaxation exercises can be the quickest and most expedient way to do it.

In addition to the Lamaze exercises described in this book, we suggest you try the visualization and breathing exercises detailed below. See which ones work for you. Incorporate them into your preparation for childbirth. Of course, you can always simply lie down for ten minutes in absolute quiet (if there is such a thing today), or listen to calming music or to a "relaxation" cassette tape. The point is to find something that works for you, and practice so that you can call upon it when the time comes.

Like many relaxation exercises, these visualization and con-trolled-breathing exercises are usually done while lying on your back, but it's possible to do them in any position that is comfortable. You can lie on your side, sit on the floor in a semireclining position, sit in a chair, or even do them in the bathtub or the shower. Just find an easy position.

Once you have established this position, try using some of the following images. Don't be surprised if you have a new favorite every day, or if, after using a couple of these a few times, you come up with your own images spontaneously. And remember, these are *only* images. You are watching them in your mind's eye. You are not *doing* anything to make them happen. The image will do the work on its own. In fact, visualization will work better if you don't interfere with any kind of forced movement.

First, scan your body. Sense any areas that feel tighter than the other areas. See if your left side feels the same as your right side and, if not, what feels different? Maybe your left arm feels longer than your right arm, maybe one side of your back makes more con-tact with the floor than the other side, maybe your shoulders feel very tight. Use this scan to become aware of any areas of your body where you have tension.

Next, check out your body part by part. One way to do this is to simply make sure that you are allowing each body part to rest com-pletely on the floor. Start at your head and go all the way down to your toes, allowing each body part, wherever it is touching the floor, to be completely supported by the floor. Or you might imagine that

- each body part is melting into the floor, or
- each body part is so heavy you couldn't possibly lift it up off the floor, or
- the floor is rising up underneath each body part to support it, or
- you are lying in the sand at the beach and allowing each body part to sink into the sand.

Images don't always have to relate to the body. Many people imagine doing something they enjoy, such as walking in the woods or on a beach. These "visions" should be as specific as possible, and should include as many sensual images as possible. It's also nice to have a partner or coach describe the scene to you as you visualize it. If you do use a coach in these exercises, he or she should describe the scene slowly, allowing you to breathe at least three times between images. Here's an example of a walk at the beach that your coach might describe to you:

Imagine you are walking down a beach. . . .

The beach is empty except for you. . . .

You can smell the salt air. . . .

A warm breeze is gently caressing your body. . . .

You hear the sea gulls calling to one another above you, and look up to count how many there are. . . .

You feel the soft, warm sand in your toes. . . .

The sun is beaming warm rays down on your body. . . .

You sit down on the beach and watch the waves rolling in and out for a long time. . . .

The importance of breathing for any and all relaxation exercises cannot be overemphasized. In fact, deep breathing by itself is a very effective relaxation technique. One breathing exercise that many people find helpful in relieving tension is to make a gentle hissing sound as you exhale. After you have "hissed," take at least three normal breaths, in and out, before you do another breath with a hiss. You might feel silly the first time you do this, but you'll quickly change your mind. Gentle hissing can relax your whole body in a very short time.

Making other sounds as you exhale is another effective relaxation technique. Singers warm up with vowel sounds, and you can exhale with vowel sounds. Try saying "U" as you exhale. Make the sound last as long as the exhalation. Do it three times in a row and then move on to saying "O" as you exhale. Continue through the vowels. Be sure to take some normal breaths, without sounds, once in a while. And whenever you use any kind of sound with your exhalations, try to keep the pitch low.

This breathing can also be incorporated with images to enhance the effectiveness of both. For example, wherever you feel tension in your body, you could imagine that your breath slowly fills that area as you inhale. Or you could imagine that the tense area is a balloon and you could watch the balloon expand as you inhale and collapse as you exhale. This is a subtle and indirect way of helping those tight muscles to relax.

Relaxation exercises can be just as effective as the Lamaze breathing exercises or any physical exercises in preparing you for giving birth. Practice them by yourself or with your coach, and try to do so every day.

It Started in Russia

Dr. Fernand Lamaze developed his childbirth preparation methods after observing the techniques used by Russian women in labor. Using the theories of conditioned response developed by Ivan Pavlov, Lamaze developed the "psychoprophylactic method" for decreasing the perception of pain or discomfort during childbirth. That phrase is a mouthful that simply means the use of distraction techniques during contractions. The method is sometimes called "mind prevention."

The Lamaze method is based on three basic breathing techniques that have been found effective during childbirth: slow-paced, moderate-paced, and pattern-paced. Originally, the method was taught very rigidly. Each breathing technique was to be used for a specific part of labor and delivery and no other. The Lamaze method of the nineties has loosened up. Women are encouraged to use the breathing techniques in the manner that is best for their individual situations. In this book, as in actual Lamaze classes, each of the three will be the subject of one intensive lesson, followed by a practice session focused on that technique (the slow technique in this chapter, moderate in the second, pattern-paced in the third). The later chapters combine the three techniques in a variety of imagined labor and delivery situations.

Before we introduce the first breathing technique, however, we must present certain Lamaze basics that pertain to all the breathing techniques and to all the practice sessions. You will probably want to refer to this section many times in the course of your pregnancy.

Use a Focal Point

An essential aspect of the Lamaze method requires picking something to focus on as an aid to concentration during labor. We refer to this as a focal point; it can be external or internal. External focal points include anything that you can literally see in the labor room. Internal focal points require your imagination. You focus on whatever images you conjure up.

Practice your breathing exercises using both kinds of focal points, because you never know what you will end up actually using during labor. Many women start out with external focal points, but find that, by the end of labor, internal focal points become more effective. A woman we know had practiced with a framed quote that normally hung in her older daughter's room. The quote read: "Faith is the substance of things hoped for, the evidence of things not seen." She thought it would be quite appropriate to use during the birth of her second child. About two hours into her labor she wanted to throw it out the window! She ended up concentrating on the panel controls on the bed.

More than likely, your focal point will come to you spontaneously during delivery. Here are some examples of both external and internal focal points that other women have used.

External Focal Points:

- Coach's face (very popular)
  Something from home, such as:
- A pair of knitted booties that a grandmother-to-be made for her new grandchild
- Pictures of family members
- Photos of calming vacation scenes
  Something in the labor room, such as:
- A light on the wall
- Flowers on the wallpaper
- A television or a clock
- A particular dot on the ceiling (very exciting)
- The holes in the ceiling tiles (One woman tried to count them with every contraction.)

Internal Focal Points:

- Images of your body at work. For example, imagine that the cervix is opening wider with each contraction.
- Images inspired by favorite music that you have brought to play in the labor room
- Images of any relaxing scene: mountains, beaches, water, etc.

Keep Your Attention on Your Breathing

The breathing that you need to use during labor and delivery requires concentration. Anything you can do to keep your attention focused on your breathing will be to your advantage. While practicing at home, turn off the TV and turn on your answering machine. Try to put everything else—hassles with the boss, the budget meeting tomorrow morning, the skirt you forgot to drop off at the cleaner's—out of your mind for these five or ten minutes that you will be practicing. Use images that are related to breathing.

Breathe Through Either Your Nose or Mouth

Try breathing *in* through your nose and *out* through your mouth, but if this doesn't work, simply breathe in whatever manner is most comfortable.

Keep Breathing

It's important not to hold your breath during practice unless you are instructed to do so. Holding your breath tenses up your body, depletes your oxygen supply, and makes the contraction much more intense. During labor, occasionally, a contraction will take you by surprise, and you may gasp and hold your breath. Sometimes, you might not even be aware that you're holding your breath, so ask your coach to make certain that you do not unconsciously hold your breath as you practice.

Clear Instructions Are Needed

Coaches, this is no time for mumbling! You need to give instructions with clarity and calmness, but also with authority.

Follow Directions

Mothers need to practice listening *carefully* to the coach and following his or her directions. Frankly, and with all preparation notwithstanding, there may come a time when you lose control and your coach's voice will be the only thing that you can "grab onto" in order to keep you going.

Practice in Different Positions

Practice your three breathing techniques while standing, walking, lying down, sitting in a rocking chair, swaying back and forth, or in any other position that you want. When the real time comes, you'll probably be changing positions constantly. Practice as many as possible now so you will have a large repertoire to choose from.

Practice Having Contractions

In the practice exercises, we will ask you to pretend that you are in labor and having contractions. We will set up "pretend" contractions and you will be asked to coordinate your breathing with the contractions. After all, the point of the breathing is to help you to get through the contraction. As you become more comfortable with your breathing techniques, it will become easier to "pretend" during practice sessions.

A word of caution: When some couples start their practice breathing they feel a little uncomfortable. Sometimes they're embarrassed or feel insecure about what they're being asked to do. Often couples get the giggles. If this happens to you and your coach, you initially might try the exercises without facing one another. But you will find that the more comfortable you become with the techniques and patterns, the easier it will be to become serious and focused.

Practice Breathing Along with Your Partner

Coaches, you need to become as familiar as possible with the breathing techniques. She will need you to breathe with her during labor. Doing the exercises right along with the expectant mother is the best way to prepare for your job, too.

Swap Roles!

An even better way to really internalize what's going on is to trade places. It's fun and enlightening for the coach, and it puts him or her on the spot about the breathing techniques. It is one thing to watch someone practice; it is another to actually participate. If your coach isn't just as familiar with the breathing techniques as you are, then that coach will never be able to assist you during labor.

Practice at Least 5 Minutes Every Day

Just as with your relaxation exercises, you can and should practice your breathing exercises anywhere—in your office, in the car, taking a bath, in bed, in the elevator, standing in line at the grocery store, or when you're just sitting around. Never mind if people stare—it's for your baby! Make a list of the breathing exercises and leave a copy on the couch, in the glove compartment, in your desk drawer—or on the desk.

Have a Paper Bag Nearby

A paper bag? Yes. You never know when you or your coach might hyperventilate. When you are practicing your breathing, as well as when you are using these breathing techniques during labor and delivery, you or your coach may feel light-headed or dizzy, or feel a tingling sensation in your hands, feet, or around your mouth. This is hyperventilation, caused by a decrease in carbon dioxide in the blood. If you should begin hyperventilating, simply breathe into your cupped hands or into a paper bag very slowly. Breathe slowly in through your nose and out through your mouth for about five minutes. This will balance your carbon dioxide supply.

Keep Track of Your Practice

As we have said, the Lamaze method calls for three types of breathing exercises. The first week of practice will incorporate the first technique and lesson, the second week should incorporate the first and second techniques, the third and subsequent weeks should incorporate all three techniques. Copy the following chart so that you can keep track of which exercises you have done during a week, and which are outstanding. If you have any problems with any of the techniques, you should make a star in that block, so that you can go back and spend more time with that technique. Circle the marks if you practiced with your partner. Here's a sample chart partially filled in:

Exercises	Slow-paced	Moderate-paced	Pattern-paced	Combinations
Week 1	X			
Week 2	X	X		X
Week 3	X	X	X	X
Week 4		X	X	X
Week 5				
Week 6				

Lamaze Breathing: Slow-paced

The first Lamaze breathing technique is slow-paced breathing. You already know how to do it because it's your natural breathing pattern when you are most relaxed, when you are lying down resting or sitting quietly reading a book. With slow-paced breathing, your chest and stomach slowly rise and fall as you inhale and exhale.

This sounds easy and natural enough, but during labor and delivery you are *not* at your most relaxed and your breathing will *not* be slow-paced of its own accord. You'll have to control your breathing. This first Lamaze breathing practice is to teach you and your coach how to incorporate slow-paced breathing during labor and delivery.

Usually, slow-paced means that you will breathe at about half your normal rate. But everyone's slow-paced breathing is a little different, so to determine what slow-paced would be for you, count your own respiration rate (the number of breaths you take in one minute) and aim to reduce that number by half with your slow-paced breathing. You will probably find that your slow-paced breathing rate is around six to nine breaths per minute. But there's no cause for alarm if yours is more or less. The important factor is cutting your respiration rate, whatever it is, in half. Try it and see what your slow-paced rate is.

Making a sound as you exhale is part of the slow-paced breathing technique. This is similar to making vowel sounds as you exhale, as described in the relaxation exercises, except with slow-paced breathing you moan as you exhale. You literally say "moan" as you exhale. The lower and deeper the pitch of your moan, the better. Get used to hearing yourself make low, groaning sounds. The thought of actually making a moaning noise may sound bizarre if not all wrong for the situation, but after a few times you will find that the moaning actually deepens your breathing and is extremely calming. It will also help keep your carbon dioxide level normal, which in turn helps prevent you from hyperventilating.

Many couples who take Lamaze classes laugh hysterically when they first try making their low-pitched sounds, but they're not laughing in the delivery room. Those low groans are great to hear during labor! Our friend Becky found herself making high-pitched

22

sounds early in her delivery. As they became higher and higher, ﹍ body tightened up worse than she could have imagined. But wi﹍ the help of her husband, who started making his own low-pitched sounds, she was able to focus and regain control.

Before we have our first practice session we must introduce one final concept, that of *deep cleansing breaths.* This type of breathing is used throughout labor and delivery, with all three Lamaze breathing techniques, and is done just as you feel a contraction beginning and again after the contraction is over. You already know how to do it, because a deep cleansing breath is simply a large sigh. It's the same type of breath you take when someone listens to your lungs through a stethoscope. It's a deep, even exchange of oxygen, inhaling through your nose and exhaling through your mouth (although it's perfectly all right to breathe exclusively through your mouth or nose). In order to guarantee this deep, even breathing, inhale to the count of ten and exhale to the count of ten as well.

So now you understand slow-paced breathing, you know your particular target rate, you can exhale with a moan, you understand how to pick a focal point, and you know what a deep cleansing breath is. It's time to put all of these skills together in a simulated labor experience. If you're not certain about a particular skill, and you may not be if this is your first experience with controlled breathing techniques, work on it further before continuing.

In this first practice session, you and your coach will do your slow-paced breathing with imagined contractions. Most contractions last around sixty seconds, so we'll ask you to use that amount of time in these practice sessions.

The instructions in every practice session are written from the coach's point of view and indicate what he or she should do or say during the session. The instructions that appear in bold face are examples of how the coach might direct the mother. They are meant simply to be a guide. As coaches practice, they begin to find their own words and style. Also, you should feel free to tell your partner if certain words or a particular way of giving instructions helps you.

1. **Sit comfortably facing each other.** Be sure you have a watch or clock with a second hand to time the contractions.

2. Begin the timing for a sixty second contraction.

Contraction begins: Take a deep cleansing breath and begin to concentrate on your focal point.

3. **Contraction is getting stronger, so now begin your slow-paced breathing. M-O-A-N with your exhalation and use your focal point.** (Coaches, be sure to breathe along with your partner.)

4. After sixty seconds: **Contraction ends. Take a deep cleansing breath.**

Slow-paced breathing can be done in any position, so now try it standing up, in this fashion:

1. Stand facing each other, and be sure your knees are just a little bent.

2. Expectant mother puts arms around the coach's neck.

3. Coach puts his or her hands on mother's waist.

4. Mother rocks her bottom slowly back and forth gently from side to side; coach can place hands on the expectant mother's hips to remind her to rock.

After you're comfortable with this new position, go through the slow-paced breathing exercise again. You'll find that the slow-paced breathing really feels comfortable in this position, especially when you let out that slow moan. Do the moan in rhythm to the rocking.

And that's it for the first breathing exercise. As you see, Lamaze work is simple and straightforward—in the classroom or while working with this book in your living room. The key is to become so confident with the breathing techniques and with each other in these comfortable, safe surroundings that you're able to transfer your skills and confidence to an altogether different environment, come crunch time.

Work Issues: Know Your Rights—The Pregnancy Discrimination Act

The unique role of women as the bearers of children has resulted in unequal treatment in employment. Before the Pregnancy Discrimination Act passed in 1978, women were commonly required to take leaves of absence at an arbitrary time before their due date. This was a very common practice for school districts, whose officials didn't think it was proper for pregnant women to teach young children once they were showing.

They also were required to return to work at an arbitrary time after delivery. If complications in pregnancy or recovery did not allow a woman to meet the mandated time frame, she often lost her job. Women were denied time off for maternity leave; it was forbidden to use vacation time or personal leave time. You were laid off.

And pregnant women were denied disability benefits during their leaves of absence. Pregnancy wasn't considered a disability, and therefore disability benefits did not apply. This treatment was blatant discrimination against women. The Pregnancy Discrimination Act (an amendment to Title VII of the Civil Rights Act of 1964) was passed to redress all pregnancy-related discriminating employment practices.

The act states that "women affected by pregnancy, childbirth, or related medical conditions shall be treated the same for all employment-related purposes, including receipt of benefits under fringe benefits programs, as other persons not so affected but similar in their ability or inability to work."

Pregnancy does not entitle you to special employment rights, but it does entitle you to the same rights as every other employee of your company. No more—but no less, either. If you are pregnant and employed, you should know that it is illegal for an employer to:

- Fire you because you are pregnant.
- Force you to go on leave (in most cases) if you are still able to do your job. The Cleveland Board of Education was ruled discriminatory in its mandatory termination provisions.
- Terminate your job on the grounds that your work will harm

25

your unborn child. Your employer may be able to mandate a pregnancy leave, modified tasks, or some other solution *if* this leave or job modification can be justified for valid work-related reasons (but it usually can't be justified) and *if* the company treats other temporarily disabled employees in the same manner. Of course, this question of suitability for a job is often a judgment call. A notable case involved a hospital that terminated a pregnant X-ray technician. She was given permission to return to her work after delivery, but she was denied her sick leave and maternity benefits. The hospital lost that case before the state Equal Employment Opportunity Commission (EEOC). The long and short of the court decisions is that the employer must play fair. Let's hope you don't have to go to court in order to get your employer to do so.

Nor may your employer:

• Mandate maternity leave for a fixed period that fails to take into account the individual needs of a specific pregnancy. (See the following chapter for a detailed section on maternity-leave issues.)
• Deny you a job because you are pregnant.
• Deny standard pregnancy-related benefits because you are not married.
• Treat your pregnancy disability differently from any other employee disability or medical condition. When you are temporarily unable to perform your job, you are entitled to the same rights to accumulate sick pay, vacation credits, and seniority as any other employee temporarily disabled by accident or illness. If employees unable to perform a task because of disability are transferred to other jobs, you have the right to be so transferred. If their jobs are held for them, your job must be held for you.
• Deny you medical or disability benefits, or leave, when the employer offers these perks for other medical conditions or disabilities. If your company policy covers an employee with a broken leg or a heart condition while he is in the hospital, it must cover your maternity expenses. (If you are a new employee, however, keep in mind that your pregnancy won't be covered if it is a "preexistent condition," which is routinely ex-

cluded from coverage. Furthermore, if your employer requires a medical examination of employees who apply for disability leave, you are likewise required to be tested for pregnancy.)

- Refuse to hold your job, or another position, for you if other temporarily disabled employees can return to their jobs after disabilities.

It is not our purpose, in this briefest of introductions to the subject of pregnancy discrimination, to serve as your attorney. We want only to alert you to problems that many other women have already encountered, and that you may, also. We want to alert you to your legal rights. Although the act was passed in 1978, it still has a lot of shortcomings for women of the 1990s. It is still ignored and therefore violated regularly—even in this society in which over 20 million working mothers struggle to nurture both their families and careers.

Many of the violations are minor, but others are quite frightening. Consider the suit that was filed against New York City by 22 presently employed and former female corrections officers who testified they were forced to have abortions or take brutal assignments in order to keep their jobs. These women won that suit; new guidelines for pregnant employees were established. But it's a disgrace that such a suit was necessary.

Let's face it: Congress didn't pass the Pregnancy Discrimination Act for the fun of it. Congress acted because it is *necessary*. Of course, having theoretical legal rights is one matter, obtaining them in the real world is another. Your status *vis-à-vis* your employer is probably much better today than it would have been twenty or even ten years ago, but many women still report unresolved problems. Immediately after a legal secretary we know announced her pregnancy, she was asked to leave, with the right to return to work after she had the baby. But this woman needed her job; she needed the money. When she went to the EEOC, her firm quickly caved in and kept her on. It's amazing that these lawyers, schooled in obtaining rights for their clients, denied them to their employee. Soured by the whole experience, this woman got another job soon after her delivery.

There is no guarantee you will win a case before the EEOC. In tough economic conditions such as these, many women may not even complain to their supervisors or to the local EEOC office for fear of the subtle or not so subtle recriminations large businesses can come up with. If a woman absolutely needs the job, she may take whatever she gets and swallow her anger and her employer's unequal treatment.

But if you feel that you are being discriminated against in the workplace due to pregnancy, and you want to take action, nothing is lost by confidentially contacting your union, should you have one, or the American Civil Liberties Union (ACLU) or the EEOC. And talk to your friends. Discrimination situations are not uncommon: the odds are excellent that someone you know has been through this before.

Taking Care of Yourself: No Time for Couch Potatoes

Regular exercise is a major factor in contributing toward a healthy and more comfortable pregnancy. Women who have exercised regularly before they were pregnant usually continue with their routine, although it may be slightly modified. Many women who have not previously exercised on any regular basis are also fitting a program into their schedule because common sense says that fitness will help prepare the body for the rigors—and they are rigors—of childbirth.

Nevertheless, some women say they just can't make the time in their busy schedules. Maybe it's true, but in our experience almost every expectant mother can find or make the time. After all, many working women have already done so. If you are a morning person, get up half an hour earlier and get your blood pumping. If you are an evening person, take the first half hour you are home from work. And if you are an in-betweener, do it on your lunch hour. A lot of downtown swimming pools are jammed with midday freestylers. The key is to establish a regular time at least three days a week. Give strong consideration to joining a health club or exercise group for pregnant women. We know women who say they just couldn't have done it without peer pressure. Whatever works.

Regular exercise will help you control your weight gain, improve your blood circulation, and help reduce water retention. It helps maintain and improve the tone of spinal, abdominal, and vaginal muscles, improving posture and helping support the extra weight. Exercise lessens fatigue, reduces tension, and promotes better sleep. Most women who exercise regularly have a more positive mental outlook and self-image throughout their pregnancy. They have fewer backaches, headaches, leg cramps, and problems with varicose veins. And exercise contributes to a more rapid postpartum recovery.

Now that you are convinced of the benefits of exercise, you want to know what kind is appropriate. To help you decide, the American College of Obstetricians and Gynecologists (ACOG) has developed guidelines for exercises during pregnancy and postpartum. Many of them pertain to exercising when you are not pregnant as well. We've summarized below ACOG's dos and don'ts.

DO:
- Exercise at least three times per week. (Woman who have led sedentary lifestyles should begin with physical activity of very low intensity and advance activity levels very gradually.)
- Take five minutes to warm up before you begin any vigorous exercise.
- Establish target heart rates in consultation with your physician.
- Monitor your heart rate during peak activity to avoid exceeding that target rate.
- Drink plenty of fluids before, during, and after exercise to prevent dehydration.
- If you exercise on the floor, get up gradually in order to avoid dizziness from temporary low blood pressure. Continue moving your legs for a brief period.
- Take time to cool down. Include some gentle stretching.
- Stop exercising and consult your doctor if any unusual symptoms appear.

DON'T:
- Exceed fifteen minutes of strenuous activity.
- Engage in competitive activities.

- Exercise vigorously in hot, humid weather.
- Exercise when you have a fever.
- Engage in "ballistic" movements (jerky, bouncy motions).
- Engage in deep flexion or extension of joints, because of connective-tissue laxity.
- Jump or engage in other jarring motions or rapid changes in direction, because of joint instability.
- Take any stretching exercise to the limit. Increased joint flexibility during pregnancy increases the risk of joint injury.
- Exercise on your back after the fourth month.
- Employ the Valsalva maneuver (used in weightlifting, forceful attempt to exhale while holding your nose and closing your mouth).

Some people in the field believe these guidelines are too general, too conservative, and not based on any research. So use these guidelines as a base. Take into account your own physical-exercise profile. Consult with your doctor as you develop your own safe and appropriate program.

Most exercises can be done within these guidelines. But let's go over some of the more popular ways to exercise and see which are appropriate for pregnant women.

Aerobics should be low-impact. Remember that the ACOG recommends no exercises in the supine position, no jerky, bouncy movements, and no deep flexions or extensions. Avoiding these activities may make most of the aerobics workout off limits to you.

Jogging is okay if you were a jogger before you were pregnant. It's not really good to start a jogging program after you're pregnant, but if you do choose to do so, start *very* slowly and with very short distances. Build distance gradually. Speed can wait until you've had your baby.

Cycling can be continued, or started safely, during pregnancy because it is not a weight-bearing activity.

Racquet sports are considered fairly safe but your game probably will have to be modified. Your coordination and balance may suffer during your pregnancy, and you can overheat more quickly.

Scuba diving, if you are already experienced, is safe if you don't exceed one atmosphere (33 feet) and limit your dive to 30 minutes.

Swimming might be the perfect exercise for pregnant women. The water has a wonderful way of making a very pregnant body feel very light. The water takes the pressure of the baby off the spine, and allows a freedom of movement impossible on dry land. A wonderful sensation!

Walking is another ideal exercise. Look around. You'll see lots of pregnant working women "putting in time" during their lunch break. Be sure to wear well-cushioned shoes.

Weightlifting, within reason, can be practiced during pregnancy with proper breathing and if the Valsalva manuever is avoided.

So: many kinds of exercise are appropriate. Some, however, should be avoided. The common ones to avoid are:

High-impact aerobics

Contact and collision sports

Basketball

Volleyball

Gymnastics

Horseback riding

Downhill and cross-country skiing

Many pregnant women join exercise classes or buy exercise tapes to work with at home. We recommend observing a class before you sign up, or previewing a tape before you buy it. Keep the ACOG Guidelines in mind. (The ACOG has also developed a pregnancy video that provides a moderate exercise program during pregnancy.) You might also consider the following criteria for judging a program:

- What are the instructor's qualifications? Is the instructor certified by IDEA (the International Dance and Exercise Association) or some other professional organization?

- Does the instructor demonstrate and explain thoroughly, or are you expected just to follow along as well as you can?
- Are the other people in the class, or on the taped program, at your level? Many videos use professional dancers; trying to keep up with them is not recommended.
- Is the speed of the exercises and the number of repetitions manageable, and is the range of motion within your limits? (A good rule of thumb: you should be able to carry on a conversation while you exercise.)
- Are you encouraged and supported to do what you are able to do, rather than to meet the expectations of the instructor?
- Are there warm-up and cool-down periods?
- Are periodic pulse checks included in the class?

Whatever exercise you choose, you should know that certain symptoms indicate that you should stop exercising *immediately*. They are:

Amniotic fluid leakage

Breathlessness

Chest pain

Dizziness

Headache

Muscle weakness

Nausea

Unusual back, hip, or pubic pain

Unusual edema

Uterine contractions

Vaginal bleeding

In each subsequent chapter of this book, one section will introduce exercises for general toning of your body, similar to exercises you would be taught in a Lamaze class. Although these exercises are excellent for muscle toning and strengthening, keep in mind that they do not provide the aerobic conditioning you would receive from activities such as walking, swimming, or bicycling. You need both types.

In this chapter we will introduce you to one exercise, the Kegel exercise, which is universally recommended and taught for childbirth preparation. It strengthens pelvic-floor muscles, promotes circulation in the perineum, and teaches you how to contract and relax these muscles voluntarily—a very important skill to acquire for labor and postpartum recovery.

If you don't know how to contract and relax your pelvic-floor muscles, you can experience it by stopping your urination midstream. We don't recommend doing this on a regular basis, but once or twice to get the idea of a pelvic-floor contraction is okay. Once you understand how to contract those muscles, you will be able to contract and relax your pelvic-floor muscles anywhere, anytime—while walking, standing in line, sitting at your desk, driving, and even during intercourse.

A variation of the simple contraction and release of the pelvic-floor muscles is the "elevator Kegel." With the elevator Kegel, you imagine that the pelvic floor is an elevator. You move upward from floor to floor as you contract the pelvic floor muscles floor by floor. At the first floor you tighten a little, the second floor a little more, and at the third floor you tighten the most. Once you're at the top, you gradually go back down, releasing the muscles little by little, floor by floor. When you reach the first floor again your pelvic floor should be as relaxed as possible.

Start doing Kegel exercises gradually. Your goal is to do fifty, three times a day. But these muscles are just like all your other muscles. If they haven't been used much previously, they tire quickly from overuse. Start out doing ten Kegel exercises (regular or elevator) three times a day. Work your way up to fifty over a period of weeks. And be sure to breathe as you do them.

Recommended Reading

General Reading

Davis, Elizabeth. *Heart and Hands: A Midwife's Guide to Pregnancy and Birth.* Berkeley, CA: Celestial Arts, 1987.

Kitzinger, Sheila. *Birth Over Thirty*. New York: Penguin, 1988.

————. *Your Baby, Your Way*. New York: Pantheon, 1987.

Panuthos, Claudia. *Transformation Through Birth*. Westport, CT: Bergin & Garvey, Greenwood, 1984.

Samuels, Mike, M.D., and Samuels, Nancy. *The Well Pregnancy Book*. New York: Summit Books, 1986.

Stoppard, Dr. Miriam. *The First Weeks of Life*. New York: Ballantine, 1989.

Weiss, Joan Solomon. *Your Second Child—A Guide for Parents*. New York: Summit Books, 1981.

CHAPTER TWO

Class 2 – Week 36

What's in This Chapter

The Beginning of the End

Lamaze Breathing: Moderate-paced

Work Issues: Maternity Leave – The "AWOL"
Dilemma

Taking Care of Yourself: Chow Down

Exercises

The Beginning of the End

Nine months is a long, long time to carry around what ends up being about 25 extra pounds, and you'll be more than ready to get
your pregnancy over with and have a real, live, squalling baby to
hold in your arms. However, when labor actually begins, you might
look back on the previous months as a veritable vacation.

Labor is a shock! Nothing prepares you for it, especially the first
time. We'll do our best in this book, but remember that, in order to
get the full flavor of the experience, "you have to be there." The
best way to be prepared is to know exactly what's coming. No surprises, ever. Forewarned is forearmed. In this chapter we get down
to the business at hand: delivering a baby.

Labor is divided into four stages. The first of these is the main
topic of this chapter, the beginning of the end. This is by far the
longest of the four stages, and includes everything that happens up
to the time you begin to push the baby out. Because so much hap-

pens during this first stage, it is often divided into three separate phases: the early, the active, and the transition phases. We'll take you through each one, step by step. But first, an overview of the situation.

If any single word sums up the experience of labor, it is *contractions*. Uterine contractions normally mark the onset of labor. They feel like a tightening of the stomach muscles, or like very strong diarrhea or flu cramps; contractions make your stomach ball up like a fist. However, the pain in a contraction comes from the cervix's changing shape, *not* from your stomach muscles. What's happening is that the uterine muscles contract when the top of the uterus becomes "irritable" and tenses. The contraction usually begins around the fallopian tubes, and may feel as if it's beginning in your back. It then spreads like a wave, moving in a downward motion, growing weaker as it reaches the bottom.

The contractions are painful, no doubt about it, but you *can* control the pain with the breathing and relaxation techniques you are learning in this book. The whole point of Lamaze breathing and the relaxation exercises is to control the pain and anxiety of the contractions. In any event, the discomfort of labor is not like having the flu or a severe stomach virus, when you get no reward for your crampy feeling and stomach spasms. With labor contractions you get a newborn baby for your cramps. It's not a bad deal, really.

As you know, your baby is surrounded and protected by amniotic fluid or, as it's commonly called, your *bag of waters*. The fluid is sealed by a membrane, which normally ruptures very early in the first stage of a normal labor. This breakage is usually one of the first signs that your labor is starting. However, there are exceptions. Some women go through their entire labor and are almost fully dilated, and their bag of waters has yet to break. Other women do have their breakage, but don't even know it. This is very possible because the breakage is not necessarily a gush of fluid, but often just a mild leak. If you have any doubt whether your bag of waters has broken, contact your doctor immediately.

When your water breaks, the fluid should be clear. You might see streaks of blood in it, which is normal, but anything more than streaks should be reported to your doctor. Amniotic fluid usually smells like semen. However, if you think that it has a foul odor, contact your doctor. If the fluid is green or any other unusual color, contact your doctor immediately. The unusual color could indicate that the baby has had a bowel movement inside the uterus, and your doctor will not want the baby to inhale this fluid during birth.

Sometimes it is necessary for your bag of waters to be broken by your doctor. Most doctors will break your bag of waters if dilation has begun and you are having heavy contractions, or if you are significantly dilated and are progressing normally except that your membranes haven't ruptured. Find out under what circumstances your doctor will rupture your membranes.

Women worry a lot about their water breaking. They worry because it means the beginning of the end. This baby you've been carrying around is finally going to be born. In all honesty, it's often a moment when women "freak out" a little, in one way or another. A woman we know had her bag of waters break when she was grocery shopping. She was embarrassed because she had leaked all over the floor. In her panic and embarrassment, she threw a glass bottle of apple juice on the same spot on the floor to hide the evidence. If you do have a big gush in public, dry yourself off and try to get home as soon as possible. As soon as you notice any fluid leaking or gushing, just contact your doctor. There's no need to panic.

A mucus plug serves as a seal between your cervix and uterus. This plug protects the uterus from infection during pregnancy. As your cervix thins and opens, this plug is loosened and released. This is called the *bloody show,* since blood vessels may rupture in the cervix and there can be blood along with the mucus. The "textbook" bloody show looks like thick mucus with some specks of bright red blood, but like everything else about childbirth, it's different for every woman. Some women may notice a bloody mucus discharge in the toilet, on the toilet paper, or on their underwear. Some women don't even know that they have lost it. But if you see blood trickling down your leg, this is too much blood, and you should contact your doctor immediately.

The first stage of labor is also called the *dilation* stage because your cervix opens to *ten* centimeters during this period. Ten centimeters is almost four inches, and this is the last time you'll read about inches in this book. The metric system is the measurement of choice in obstetrics.

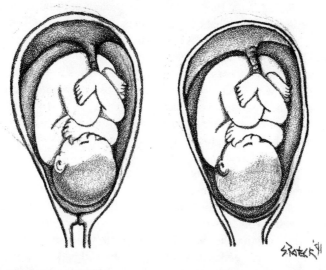

Effacement or Dilation   **Effacement and Dilation**

Dilation of the cervix—the opening of the cervix—usually begins to occur just before you go into labor. You may even dilate one or two centimeters during the last month of pregnancy. This is completely normal, and nothing to worry about.

Your cervix also has to thin out as well as dilate. This thinning out is called *effacement.* In first pregnancies, it usually takes place before dilation begins, but it occurs simultaneously in repeat births. There is no external sign of effacement. It is determined only by an internal exam, and it is measured in percentages. Your doctor might tell you that you are 80 percent effaced just before you are ready to push. The percentage indicates how much your cervix has thinned out. The higher the percentage the better, 100 percent being the ultimate number.

False Labor

Most first-time mothers are not sure if they are having true contractions or false labor. In fact, the most common question of women pregnant for the first time is probably, "How do I know if I'm in labor?" (You won't have any doubts the second time around.) The real thing is generally accompanied by those very clear signs discussed above. Your water breaks and you have a bloody show. Also, your cervix starts to dilate, but only your nurse or doctor can tell you this. In true labor, the contractions are strong and consistent.

False labor may fool you initially but probably not for long. To begin with, the contractions are irregular, unlike true labor contractions. False labor contractions tend not to follow any consecutive pattern. If you start timing your contractions and find that you have one or two within the first hour, then nothing the next hour, you are most likely dealing with a false alarm.

With false labor there isn't a noticeable bloody show, which is another indication that this isn't the real thing. If you are checked by your doctor and told that there isn't any effacement or any dilation of the cervix—false labor. And, of course, the best, surest sign of false labor is . . . no baby! A woman we know experienced really deceitful false labors with two of her four children. They were good fakes, but with the second false alarm, she knew to wait it out and see what would happen. Most first-time mothers are so excited with the first sign of anything happening that they want to rush to the hospital. This is quite understandable, but a waste of energy and emotional strength if it turns out to be a false alarm. Put the clock on the first contractions. Check for the bloody show. If you conclude you are being teased by a false labor, just sit in a warm tub. Your contractions will probably stop. If you can, try to sleep (but not in the tub).

Preterm Labor

A word about labor that occurs before the thirty-seventh week of gestation. Lamaze classes and the discussions in this book assume a full-term pregnancy (approximately 280 days, or 40 weeks), or nearly so. But this is not always the case. If you feel as if you are having contractions—real contractions—many weeks before your official due date, contact your doctor. Most doctors will attempt to stop preterm labor by placing the mother on bedrest accompanied by medication to stop contractions.

Phases of the First Stage

You are not in false labor: your contractions are regular, your water has broken, you are dilated to some degree. Certainly, the first stage of labor has begun. Your contractions become faster and more intense, your cervix completes most of its dilating, and you have more and more work to do. As we stated earlier, this stage is broken down into three smaller phases: early, active, and transition. Here's a closer look at each one.

Early Phase

The early phase is marked by those initial signs discussed above. Your water breaks, your contractions start (usually about 4 to 5 minutes apart and lasting between 30 and 45 seconds), and your cervix dilates from 0 to 4 or 5 cm. This early phase is the happy, excited, "we finally made it!" phase. It may also be the easiest. You will probably not be terribly uncomfortable, and you won't have to focus on what you're doing as much as you will later. This phase generally lasts 7 or 8 hours. But remember, every delivery is different and the time for any stage can vary drastically.

However, some women experience *prodromal labor* during the early stage. Prodromal labor is an irregular labor that can last for days on end unless something is done to curtail it. Neither you nor your doctor wants this pattern to continue if you are nauseated, vomiting, or becoming exhausted. Going into the final stages of labor dog-tired and sleepless is really tough. If you notice a prodromal pattern setting in, get in a warm shower and twirl your nipples. This may seem like some of kind of bizarre old wives' tale, but in fact it can produce a spurt of oxytocin, which will help stimulate contractions of the uterus, and might start labor.

How to Manage the Early Phase:

- Stay home and try to relax. Try to calm yourself and pass the time by watching a movie or visiting with a family member. This is a great time to talk to your coach and enjoy each other's company. It may be the last time you'll have real peace and quiet for some time.

- Keep track of your contractions. Check to see how long each one lasts, how often the contractions occur, and how strong they are. (Make sure that you have a watch with a second hand for timing the contractions.) To find out how long your contractions are, jot down when a contraction begins and when it ends. Easy subtraction gives you the answer.

  To calculate how often you're having contractions, time from the beginning of one contraction to the beginning of the next contraction. Again, write down both numbers and do your math.

- Call your doctor when your contractions have been as close as five minutes apart for at least one hour.
- Try using your slow-paced breathing with the contractions encountered during this phase.
- When your bag of waters breaks, check the color and odor of the fluid. Once your membranes have ruptured, take showers (*not* baths, because of potential infection).
- Sometimes women experience a terrible backache, caused by the baby's pressing against the sacrum and coccyx. It's uncomfortable, certainly, but another good sign that your labor is moving along. If you are experiencing a backache, pelvic-tilt exercises will relieve some of the discomfort. Also, having the coach massage your lower back is relaxing, and he or she can roll a tennis ball around on your lower back. Use of the tennis ball helps keep the coach's hands from becoming sore and tired.
- If you get the shakes, which is common during labor, get your paper bag and begin breathing into it.

Active Phase

The second phase of the first stage of labor is called the active phase, because it is just that. It generally lasts 3 to 5 hours, during which time the contractions are more intense and much closer together. They will be about 3 to 4 minutes apart and last 50 to 70 seconds. Your cervix dilates to 5 to 7 cm.

Now is when your work really begins. And from this point on, no one really knows when the baby will emerge. Delivery could be hours away, or it could happen very rapidly. You will feel much more comfortable and relaxed if you are at the hospital or birthing center, with your nurse only a call button away. If you are having a home birth, this is the time to settle in with a quiet environment.

How to Manage the Active Phase:

- You will need to concentrate much more during this phase. Try moderate-paced breathing (see page 52). Some women continue with the slow-paced breathing during this phase, but many switch to the moderate-paced or a combination of the two. Having your coach breathe with you will help keep you on track.

- Definitely change positions often. Changing positions will help you pass the time, keep your mind focused on something other than the contractions, and allow you to be as comfortable as you can be. Walking, standing, rocking in a standing position or in a rocking chair, sitting on hands and knees in a "crawling" position, lying on your side, standing and leaning forward on a bedside table, sitting and leaning forward with support from your coach, and kneeling and leaning forward on a chair or your coach: all are good positions to experiment with.

- Try taking a shower. Many women find "hydrotherapy" relaxing. One woman we know stood in the shower her entire labor and held on to the shower handle for dear life. Her husband stood with her and felt like a "prune" when it was time to deliver. Even her doctor examined her in the shower!

- Make sure that you are taking some form of liquid, even if you don't feel like it, to keep from dehydrating. Suck on ice chips if you can't get anything else down. (This ploy seems to be a standard feature of movie and television deliveries.)

- Keep cool. You'll be hot and perspiring from all of your hard work. Let your coach cool you off with a washcloth dipped in cold water. Use a fan.

- If you are vomiting, and you may be because of the riot of hormones coursing through your body, ask for some glycerin swabs to moisten your mouth and lips.
- Ask for medication if you need it. Traditionally, medication will be given at approximately 4 to 5 cm of dilation. In the nineties, doctors are more willing to give you medication whenever you request it, regardless of how dilated you are, but there are always extenuating circumstances. They don't believe you should be in uncontrollable pain any time during your labor and delivery.

Transition

During this last phase of the first stage of labor, your cervix reaches maximum dilation, and your contractions, which are much more intense now, come every 1 to 2 minutes and last 80 to 90 seconds. By the end of this transition, all systems are "go" for pushing. The transition phase usually lasts anywhere from 1/2 to 2 hours.

You may feel anxious and worried that this will never end. It will! You may also become slightly irrational and lose control. Don't worry about it—you won't be the first! Teamwork with your coach will help get you through this phase. And, if you've practiced your breathing responsibly, this is the phase where it pays off.

How to Manage the Transition Phase:

- Keep changing positions, just as you did in the active phase.
- Let yourself rest between contractions. Try any of your relaxation techniques. Some women actually fall asleep between contractions, which is a great help to your stamina.
- Focus on your breathing. Focus on your breathing. Focus on your breathing. This is an indispensable mantra.
- Let your coach help you. If you can tell your coach what you need, do so. If you're losing control, pass the control to this stalwart. He or she is fully prepared to accept it.
- Save your pushing for later. At 8 to 10 cm, you can be very tired and discouraged, and you might be tempted to start push-

ing before you are actually ready to push. If you begin pushing too early, you can have swelling in the cervix, which can make a vaginal delivery very difficult.

At this point we break off the story, under the assumption that this is enough for one reading session. We want you to learn this information, not gag on it. The delivery saga continues in the next chapter. Take a break, turn the page—do some breathing!

Lamaze Breathing: Moderate-paced

Moderate-paced breathing is the second type of Lamaze breathing you need to learn. It's much faster and shallower than the slow-paced breathing you learned in Chapter One. With moderate-paced breathing, you inhale and exhale with short, light, shallow breaths, just as when you are trying to catch your breath after strenuous exercise.

Obviously, your respiration rate will be faster than with the slow-

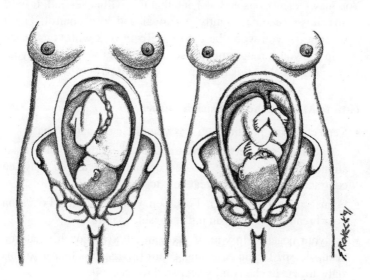

Well-flexed Position   **Posterior Presentation**

paced breathing, but your rate shouldn't exceed two times your normal respiration rate. The maximum respiration rate will be around 24 breaths per minute. This next statement may sound contradictory, but it isn't: within the faster breathing rate, always breathe as slowly as you can. Counting 1–2–3 between breaths will assure this, and will therefore help prevent hyperventilation.

Moderate-paced breathing can be done in several ways. Here are two versions; practice both.

Version 1: ha 1–2–3

1. Inhale slowly and easily.
2. Sound a "ha" as you exhale (soft, gentle puff).
3. Count to 3 before you inhale again. Actually say the numbers 1–2–3 out loud.

Version 2: The second version is a 3-breath pattern. It sounds like: "hee, ha, who," with short breaks or pauses in between. Try it.

1. Inhale slowly and easily.
2. Exhale with a "hee" sound.
3. Inhale slowly and easily.
4. Exhale with a "ha" sound.
5. Inhale slowly and easily.
6. Exhale with a "who" sound.

When you can do both versions without having to read the instructions, you're ready for this chapter's breathing exercises, which incorporate both slow-paced and moderate-paced breathing techniques with simulated contractions.

Starting with this practice session, when it's possible, place an ice bag on your wrist or have your coach pinch your Achilles tendon as a simulation of beginning of a contraction. Also, with this session, have your coach vary the length and pace of contractions for you. In this way your coach will simulate the different phases of labor so you will be able to handle slow contractions as well as the fast and hard ones.

(As in the practice session in Chapter One, the instructions and the statements within quotations are for the coach.)

1. Pinch partner's Achilles tendon to indicate beginning of the contraction.

   Begin timing the contraction.

   Take a deep cleansing breath or two. Remember, they're like huge sighs.

2. After 25 seconds:

   The contraction is becoming stronger. Be sure you have your focal point and begin your slow-paced breathing.

   Begin breathing with your partner.

3. After 30 seconds:

   Contraction is peaking—begin your moderate-paced breathing. Let's do it together. It's inhale, then ha 1–2–3. Inhale and ha 1–2–3. . . .

   (Version 2: Inhale hee, inhale ha, inhale who.)

4. After 45 seconds:

   Contraction is subsiding, return to your slow-paced breathing.

5. After 1 minute:

   It's over. Take another deep cleansing breath or two.

We divided that exercise above into four equal segments with the peak of the contraction coming 30 seconds after it began. Needless to say, not all contractions (perhaps even none) will follow this pattern. So now go back and repeat this same exercise many times, but vary the length of the contractions and when they peak. With this repetition, use version 2 of the moderate-paced breathing.

You have now mastered the second of the three Lamaze breathing techniques.

Work Issues: Maternity Leave — The "AWOL" Dilemma

One immediate issue that faces the pregnant working woman is the question of a leave of absence from work. It has been our experience that many women believe federal law *entitles* them to maternity leave, perhaps as a function of the Pregnancy Discrimination Act we discussed in the previous chapter.

Unfortunately, this is not correct. The United States stands alone as an affluent, industrialized country that fails to provide even minimal support to mothers. In Europe, five months following childbirth is typical maternity leave. Although the Family and Medical Leave bill of 1991 now before Congress would mandate maternity leave, there is no guarantee it will be passed or signed into law by the President. This legislation guarantees workers up to 12 weeks of unpaid leave for the birth of a child *or* a family illness. It was passed in 1990 by Congress, but President Bush vetoed it. He has said he will do so again unless the "family illness" clause is deleted. Forty states have stepped into the vacuum and instituted some kind of family-leave policy, and it's fairly likely that sometime in the not too distant future all women will be legally entitled to maternity leave. But right now federal regulations do *not* guarantee this right, and state regulations are not uniform.

What is guaranteed is your right to a *disability* leave *if* your company has disability leave for other medical situations. This distinction between a maternity and a disability leave is very important, and we will explain it more fully in a moment. But first things first:

Does Your Company Have a Leave Policy At All?

When you find out you are pregnant, or perhaps even when you are planning to become pregnant, find out about your company's policy. If you are looking for a job and planning to have a family, check to see if any child-care benefits are included in the company's fringe-benefit package. (Planning before pregnancy pays off if your company has no policy whatsoever, and you fear you might lose your job or be in for major hassles. You might take this Neanderthal attitude into account when timing your pregnancy.)

If yours is a large company, the personnel office will have the facts, in writing, usually in the employees' handbook. However, these handbooks are not always up-to-date. Check to make certain that the policy hasn't changed. If it has changed, you would be wise to get these changes in official written form.

Discuss any ambiguous language in the policy with the appropriate corporate officer. You will find it helpful to talk with other women in the firm who have had babies fairly recently, to determine if their actual experience matches the official policy. These mothers can tell you whether obtaining your rights is easy or a struggle, whether you are likely to suffer subtle discrimination regardless of what the policy says. Unless you are extremely confident of your company's goodwill, check things out from every possible angle. Perhaps you feel we exaggerate the possible complications. We don't.

The smaller your employer, the less likely it is to have an official policy. Fortune 500 companies will have them, and they will provide for maternity leave, but the small shop with six or even sixty employees is another matter. Maybe no one with your company has even taken maternity leave before. A scary situation, perhaps, but look at it this way: you are in a position to negotiate a deal that can become an enlightened policy that will benefit other women in the future. On the other hand, if your firm has no official policy but other women have taken leaves and negotiated their own deals, these may now serve as an unwritten policy and you may feel stuck with a poor situation.

Be prepared. Before you approach your employer, find out if other women have taken leave; if they have, find out what happened. Decide whether you can live with this. If you can't, marshal your arguments before you sit down with the boss. Know your rights.

What Kind of Leave Does Your Company Provide?

In order to comply with the Pregnancy Discrimination Act discussed in the previous chapter, companies that offer maternity leave do so as a form of medical disability. In fact, the law decrees that maternity leave must be accepted as a medical disability if the company has a disability policy. All large companies will have such a policy; small ones, not necessarily.

In addition, a few very progressive companies offer *parental* leave as distinguished from maternity leave. Parental leave is usually offered in addition to maternity/disability leave and, according to the EEOC, it must be available to both males and females, if either. Parental leave usually includes leave for birth or the adoption of a baby or caring for ill dependents. More on this subject in a moment.

Is Your Leave Paid or Unpaid?

Most leaves are unpaid, but some, mostly at major corporations, are paid. AT&T, as one example, allows six weeks' paid maternity leave and up to a year's unpaid parental leave. But even unpaid maternity leaves are eligible for disability insurance because they are carried "on the books" as medical disability leaves. Disability insurance will pay a percentage of your salary for a specified period of time. You will have to apply for it.

To apply for disability benefits, contact the Employment Development Department (EDD). They will send you an application form and booklet explaining how and when to send in the completed form. Your doctor will have to sign the form acknowledging that you are unable to work, and stating when he expects you to be able to return. Once you and your doctor have filled out the EDD form, you can mail it in, and you will receive your disability checks in approximately two weeks.

If you need information regarding unpaid pregnancy disability leave, or if your company is giving you a difficult time on this subject, contact the Department of Fair Employment and Housing (DFEH).

How Much Time Are You Allowed?

This varies drastically. It may be from the minimal (and absurd) two weeks to as much as one year. Find out. Read the fine print. The

United States Postal Service offers a thirteen-week unpaid maternity leave—a fairly standard policy for government employees. Pacific Gas and Electric is in the forefront with its maternity-leave policy, which offers six months, unpaid, for birth, adoption, or legal guardianship, with a "same job" guarantee on return. In addition to those six months, mothers can take another additional six months with the stipulation that they are not guaranteed their same positions, but only some positions if there are vacancies.

It should come as no surprise that executives appear to have an advantage negotiating a reasonable leave, due to their elevated status and seniority in the company. The wave of the future may turn out to be a sliding scale for maternity leave, based on seniority and length of time with the company.

How Much Time Do You Need?

How much time off your company allows and how much you want or require may be very different indeed. Only you can decide how much time you need. In making your decision, you will want to consider how long you can effectively do your job before delivery, how long you can be gone without losing effectiveness on your return, and, most important of all, how long you want to stay home with your baby. The final answer—how much leave to take or at least request—is not always easy to determine.

Many, perhaps most, women want to work as long as possible during their pregnancy, if there are no complications, thus saving as much time as possible for time at home with the newborn. As we discussed in Chapter One, years ago women were often forced to stop work at a certain point in their pregnancy. Now women are able to work right until they go to the hospital, should they want to, and many do. Others need to take time off before their due dates because of complications in their pregnancies. If this extended predelivery time is medically mandated by your physician, your company is required to provide it, just as it would provide leave for any other medical disability.

Women also differ on how much time they want to take off after their babies are born. Some are ready to go back after a few weeks, but for others a few months is not enough. Many women love their work and may even feel a twinge of guilt if they don't want to avail themselves of the full time allowed by their company. We can't imagine the mother who would not want two measly weeks of leave, but we know many women who would truly miss their work after several months. They miss their work and then, upon returning to work, miss their children.

In short, you may have somewhat contradictory emotions that cannot be neatly reconciled. But you will, in any event, have to make a decision, and you will have to do so *before* you go on leave. Almost all employers will want to know when you plan to return, and this is a fair enough request on their part. Some employers will go along with an informal, modified leave. Our friend Carol's law firm offered twelve weeks' maternity leave. For a variety of reasons, she did not want to be gone that long, but she did want shorter hours for the twelve weeks. The law firm was happy to have her part-time services.

If You Need More Time, Is Your Company Flexible?

Your company allows you two weeks, but you want four. Or your company gives you six weeks, but you want eight. If you find yourself in this situation, and you may very well, you may be stuck with the prescribed amount of time. But you may also have several options for reconciling the difference. Many companies will allow you to use vacation time or accumulated sick days in order to extend your maternity-disability leave. Other companies—mainly some of the very large ones—will allow you to extend the basic leave of absence with a special maternity leave. And there may be other possibilities. Check with other women in your company and see what they have arranged.

When and How Do You Make Your Request?

The question of announcing a pregnancy is one of the diciest that many working women confront. How will your boss handle the

51

news? Will she or he take you and your career less seriously? Will your coworkers do the same? Will you have hassles negotiating a suitable leave? These are often justifiable concerns, but just as often they turn out to be worry over nothing. We suggest you carefully pick the time and the place for the announcement and see what develops.

Timing is important. Consider if you are in line for a promotion, a raise, or have a major business trip planned. You don't need to negotiate your leave of absence as soon as you find out you are pregnant, but give your employer and yourself enough time to prepare. Most women tend to wait until the very last minute, when they are just about to show. Women over thirty-five years often want to wait for the results of amniocentesis. It's your call, of course, but do consider the specifics of your job and how your departure, even temporarily, will affect the work of your coworkers. How long will be required to find someone to replace you, if this is necessary? Will this replacement require training from coworkers? Rare is the job in which you can, without nasty repercussions, announce on Monday your intention of departing on Friday for four months of maternity leave. This is just poor form.

Your boss may not be the first person you want to tell that you're pregnant, but you don't want her or him to find out through the grapevine, either. And he or she *will* find out through the grapevine if you delay very long. When you're ready to disclose your pregnancy, be sure your boss is near the top of the list. Get negotiations off on the right footing.

The way to request a leave officially varies from company to company. We can't offer advice on this. Check the policy. But we can tell you to be prepared when you make your request. *And put it in writing.* Know the specific dates you want to leave and return. If you want to work part time, and this is an option, be clear about the days and hours you would work. Build flexibility into your request. Check the calendar of upcoming events at your company.

Let's take the hypothetical case of the CPA whose due date is April 25. She has six weeks of maternity leave coming, and the ideal for her would be two weeks before the baby comes and four weeks after. But from her accounting firm's perspective, for obvious reasons, the latest possible departure date would be best—something after April 15, when the tax rush is over. If this woman likes her job and her employer, it would behoove her to be as flexible as possible and change her schedule. Situations you are more likely to encounter would involve important meetings, conventions, production deadlines, and the like.

Decide whether you want or need to stay involved with your job while you are on leave. Many women want to be completely removed from their jobs, while others may be required to stay involved at some level. Lawyers would probably be in this latter category, dealing as they must with a steady stream of paperwork. Don't wait until the last minute to work out keep-in-touch details with bosses and coworkers.

Consider how your workload can be delegated. If a temporary replacement will be hired, will it be necessary or appropriate for you to interview candidates? Train the individual hired?

You might think that such questions are automatically resolved early and efficiently in the well-run businesses of America, but if you check around, you'll hear plenty of stories about last-minute chaos. And inevitably, some or most of the negative fallout from these problems will be laid on your doorstep.

When you make your request for a leave of absence, try to obtain a specific date by which you will know if it has been approved. If that day comes and goes without an answer, it's your responsibility to follow up on the request. This is especially important if you work in a large company burdened with a seemingly endless bureaucracy. Requests get lost, personnel can change, and you find yourself a week before your hoped-for departure with a request that hasn't even been approved.

Budgeting for Maternity Leave

It would be nice to know that you have already done some financial planning for the upcoming blessed event. However, the majority of parents do not plan ahead, so we'll offer a few gratuitous observations and pose some obvious but sometimes overlooked questions that you need to answer.

First, what's this baby going to cost? We can't tell you because the answer depends on your standard of living and varies greatly from doctor to doctor, hospital to hospital, state to state. Check with friends who live about as you do, and who have children. They'll know the answer.

How much of your medical expenses will have to come out of pocket? This one is easy enough to figure. How much time can you afford for an unpaid leave of absence, if your company offers one? Again, only you know the answer. An ideal step, for those who can afford to do so, is to sit down with a financial planner who can lay out a twelve-month budget. A number of books on the market can also give you the charts and graphs you'll need for this planning. But, frankly, it's hard to do all this. Have the baby, and it will cost what it costs: that seems to be the attitude of most new parents. Okay, but a little advance thinking might indicate that a six-month leave, most of it unpaid, is just beyond your means. Or you might realize that you can afford more time than you would have guessed. Our main tip on budgeting is to do just that: budget. The physical business of delivering the baby may seem easy in comparison.

What About Men?

A growing number of men want to spend time with their newborn babies, but few men are able to do so. As we said, some companies now have "gender-free" parental leave policies. Lotus, the computer software company, offers one month's *paid* parental leave, but this is highly unusual. "Paternity leave" for men is usually a well-kept secret. In many companies there is an unwritten rule: real men don't do it. A man's commitment to his job is questioned; his career can stall. Even men who only want a week off after the births of their babies often take it under the guise of vacation or illness. Any association at all with "maternity leave" can be a detriment to their careers. Of course, this is nothing new to women!

Nevertheless, a small percentage of men are taking paternity leave. The need to spend time with their babies outweighs the unspoken penalties. It is usually a conscious decision to jump from the fast track onto the daddy track. However, it may also make economic sense. Although in most two-career couples the woman earns less, some women earn more than their spouses. A logical option here is for the lower-paid husband to take the unpaid leave. (But can his ego handle it? That's another issue.) In a few situations, husbands take the longer leave because their companies have a better leave policy. And some adroit couples use staggered leaves—first one, then the other—in order to avoid as long as possible placing their babies in child care.

Taking Care of Yourself: Chow Down

Pregnancy is the time when many women finally learn to eat well. This is a time when you *must* be good to your body, so that you will be good to your baby. If you are a junk-food junkie, you'd better reevaluate and modify your diet. A little junk every once in a while isn't too bad, but a steady diet of the stuff is not recommended for anyone.

Most doctors and nutritionists recommend three meals a day and three snacks a day for pregnant women. Eating six times a day may seem outrageous to you, but it seems to work best.

Whole-grain or enriched breads are preferred, and it is recommended that you choose cereals with fiber and whole grain. Avoid all sugared cereals. Eat whole fruits rather than drinking fruit juices, unless they are pure fruit juices. Avoid fruit drinks that have a high content of water and sucrose, juices with only 10 percent fruit, or juices with added sugar.

Avoid alcohol. Up until the seventies, it was thought that alcohol had no effect on an unborn baby. Now we know that alcohol crosses the placenta freely and attains blood levels in the baby similar to those in the mother, and it has a toxic effect on the developing baby. Fetal alcohol syndrome, a substantial risk for babies, retards the unborn baby both mentally and physically, causes developmental delays and various congenital malformations of the head, face, skeleton, and heart. A recent study shows a direct relationship between spontaneous abortion and drinking. Even an occasional binge or two drinks per day can have severe side effects, such as low birth weight and poor muscle tone.

Avoid caffeine. Most people relate caffeine to coffee and tea, but it's also found in chocolate, many soft drinks, and iced tea. Caffeine is a stimulant that increases the heartbeat and metabolic rate, and causes a rise in epinephrine (adrenaline), which reduces the blood flow to the uterus, which reduces the flow of oxygen and nutrients to the baby. The Food and Drug Administration has warned pregnant women to reduce their levels of caffeine during pregnancy. Doctors prefer that you avoid it altogether by switching to decaffeinated coffee and tea (and only two cups per day, because decaffeinated still contains trace amounts), and avoid caffeinated soft drinks.

If your office has coffee and tea flowing freely all day, as most do, it's easy to get in the habit of having a few cups to keep going, especially when the fatigue of pregnancy is an inevitable occurrence. Try to wean yourself of this habit by cutting down to two cups per day, then one cup, and then to decaffeinated coffee. If you feel tired during the day, try walking or other exercises.

Most nutritionists and doctors agree that even women who eat good, balanced meals should receive supplemental prenatal vitamins. The need for these vitamins is not universally agreed upon, but the majority would recommend them.

Talk to your doctor or a nutritionist about your diet. You may not think you need a special diet, but she or he may see things differently. For example, if you are vomiting, have had a pregnancy less than a year earlier, have a poor obstetrical history of any kind, have failed to gain ten pounds by the twentieth week, or have undue emotional stress, specific dietary changes may be recommended. These will not be drastic or overly regimented, but specific enough so you will eat what you need.

If you are a vegetarian, you can safely continue your vegetarianism throughout pregnancy. But you must plan your diet carefully, possibly with the help of a nutritionist or registered dietician, and you should add supplements at certain times. The more restricted your diet, the more carefully planned it must be: the strict vegetarian who avoids all foods of animal origin needs to plan more carefully than the ovo-lacto vegetarian (who does eat eggs and milk).

These cautionary remarks do not mean that you should spend your pregnancy obsessing over the nutrient content of everything on your plate, but some early planning will keep your days of waiting worry-free. Plan your diet before you get too far into your pregnancy, or prior to conception if you can.

If you are not placed on any special diet by your doctor, you can use the list below to help you plan and balance your meals. The list includes suggested number of daily servings in the four food groups, plus recommended serving sizes for pregnant adults, for lactating adults, and for pregnant teenagers.

Protein-Rich Foods

Provide: Protein, iron, thiamin, niacin

Essential for: Tissue building

Serving size:
Beef, veal, organ meats,
   lamb, poultry, pork (2 oz.)
Fish and shellfish (2 oz.)
Peanut butter (1/4 cup)
Cottage cheese (1/2 cup)
Nuts and seeds
Eggs (2 medium)
Tofu (1 cup)
Beans (1 cup): lima, kidney, soy,
   navy, mung, black, pea

Daily servings:
Pregnant adult 3–4 servings
Lactating adult 3–4 servings
Pregnant teen 3–4 servings
Lactating teen 3–4 servings

Protein Snacks: Peanut butter, nuts, and seeds (1/2 cup)

Milk and Milk Products

Provide: Calcium, protein, vitamins A and D, phosphorus, zinc, and magnesium

Essential for: Healthy bones and teeth

Serving Size:
Nonfat, low-fat, or
  whole milk (1 cup)
Yogurt, plain (1 cup)
Soymilk or tofu (1 cup)
Pudding/custard (1 cup)
Nonfat milk powder (1/3 cup)
Cottage cheese (1 1/2 cups)
Cheese (1 1/2–2 oz.)
Ice cream (1 3/4 cups)

Daily servings:
Pregnant adult 4 servings
Lactating adult 5 servings
Pregnant teen 5 servings
Lactating teen 6 servings

Snacks: Milk, cottage cheese, yogurt

Vitamin-A-Rich Fruits and Vegetables

Provide: Iron, folacin, vitamins A, E, C, K, and fiber

Essential for: Soft skin, good eyesight

Serving Size:
Apple or banana (1)
Apricots, nectarines,
  plums (2)
Dates (3), prunes (4)
Pumpkin (1/4 cup)
1 cup raw or 1 cup cooked:
  broccoli, zucchini, spinach,
  potato, cauliflower, yams,
  carrots, cabbage, corn,
  chicory, endive, escarole,
  greens (beet, collard, mustard),
  summer or winter squash

Daily servings:
Pregnant adult 1–2 servings
Lactating adult 1–2 servings
Pregnant teen 1–2 servings
Lactating teen 1–2 servings

Vitamin-A-Rich Snacks: V-8 juice, banana, apple

Vitamin-C-Rich Fruits and Vegetables

Provide: Vitamin C and fiber

Essential for: Connective tissue and resistance to infection

Serving size:
Orange or tangerine (1)
Mango or papaya (1)
Grapefruit, cantaloupe,
  or strawberries (1/2 cup)
Pineapple or tomato juice
  (1 1/2 cups)
Broccoli (1 stalk)
Cabbage or cauliflower (3/4 cup)
Brussels sprouts (3–4)
Greens: Collard, kale, or mustard (3/4 cup)

Daily servings:
Pregnant adult 2+ servings
Lactating adult 2+ servings
Pregnant teen 2+ servings
Lactating teen 2+ servings

Vitamin-C-Rich Snacks: Orange, grapefruit, tomato

Bread, Cereal, and Grain Foods

Provide: B vitamins, iron, trace minerals, and fiber

Essential for: Healthy blood, nerve tissue, and bowel function

Serving Size:
Bread (1 slice)
Roll, muffin, biscuit, tortilla (1)
Pasta/noodles or rice (1/2 cup)
Cooked cereals (1/2 cup)
Dry cereals (3/4 cup)
Wheat germ (1 tablespoon)

Daily servings:
Pregnant adult 4 servings
Lactating adult 4 servings
Pregnant teen 4 servings
Lactating teen 4 servings

Snacks: Whole-grain muffin or popcorn

Fats and Oils

Provide: Vitamins A and D, linoleic acid, calories

Essential for: Energy, healthy skin

Serving size: (3 teaspoons per day total; to be used in moderation)
Butter, margarine, mayonnaise
Cream cheese, whipped cream
Avocado, nuts, fatty cheeses
Vegetable oils, cooking fats
Prepared salad dressings

Daily servings:
Pregnant adult 1 serving
Lactating adult 1 serving
Pregnant teen 1 serving
Lactating teen 1 serving

Snacks: Nuts, cheese cubes

Exercises

Our aim in each "Exercise" section of this book is to improve or maintain your general muscle tone and flexibility. While we do not specify which muscle groups benefit from specific exercises—too technical for our purposes—special emphasis will be placed on exercises to strengthen your pelvic floor and your abdominal muscles. Here, we would like to add a word of caution about your abdominals. Many pregnant women experience *recti diastasis,* which is separation of the rectus abdominis muscle. Your abdominal muscles are softening because of hormonal changes and stretching to accommodate your expanding uterus. It is important to avoid exercises or positions, such as double leg lifts and sit-ups, that might encourage more separation of the abdominal muscles. And, of course, check with your doctor if you have any question abut the condition of your abdominals or exercises that you should or should not do.

We would also like to add another word of caution: if you are on bedrest, *absolutely* do not attempt any of these exercises. In fact, just skip all the exercise sections so you won't even be tempted. If you aren't on bedrest, proceed.

In each chapter, the exercises are organized by starting positions. They build slowly as you progress from chapter to chapter, but feel free to mix them up. You'll probably have favorites that you'll want to do every day.

As you do the exercises, keep the following in mind:

- These exercises should feel good to do. While doing them, pay attention to your body and how it feels while you are doing the exercises. The "no pain, no gain" philosophy does not apply here.
- These exercises can be done as slowly as you need to do them. There's no instructor cracking a whip to make you keep up with the rest of the class. Take the time to do each exercise fully.
- The exercises should be done within your range of movement. For example, if the instructions ask you to turn your head to the left, it's not necessary to crank your head all the way around until your nose is over your shoulder. Moving your head an inch to the right is fine. You can increase your range of movement gradually, but you can also keep in mind that bigger is not necessarily better. Small movements are often more beneficial than large ones.

  In particular, your belly may limit how high you can lift your leg. Use your common sense and adjust the exercise accordingly.
- There is no specified number of "reps" for each exercise. Some you may only want to repeat two or three times. Others you may want to do as many as eight to ten times. Twenty is probably too many repetitions for any of these exercises. Start with two or three and build from there.
- Be sure that you are breathing throughout each exercise. Many exercise books will instruct you when you inhale and exhale during an exercise. We suggest you experiment with your breathing. You decide when you inhale and exhale. See what works best for you.

Sitting

1. Starting Position: Sit with your legs folded in front of you or with the soles of your feet touching in front of you.
- Rock side to side, from one hip to the other. Feel yourself rock-

ing from one sitz bone to the other. (Your sitz bones are actually the part of your pelvis that you sit on. If you're not sure where they are, place your hands underneath your buttocks while you are sitting. The bones that you feel squashing your hands are your sitz bones.)

You can either let your hands rest on your knees or use them to help push you from one side to the other.

2. Starting Position: Same as 1. (Sit with your legs folded in front of you or with the soles of your feet touching in front of you.)

• Rock forward and backward on your pelvis. Imagine rocking from your tailbone to your pubic bone as you shift back and forth.

3. Starting Position: Same as 1. (Sit with your legs folded in front of you or with the soles of your feet touching in front of you.)

• Move your pelvis so that you draw an imaginary diamond with it. Shift forward to your pubic bone, then shift diagonally back to your left sitz bone, next back to your tailbone, followed by a shift diagonally forward to your right sitz bone, and finally shift to your pubic bone. Repeat several times and then reverse directions.

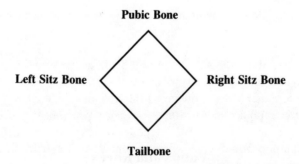

• Move your pelvis so that you draw a circle instead of a diamond. You can imagine that you are tracing the hours on the face of a clock. Repeat several times and be sure to circle clockwise and counter-clockwise.

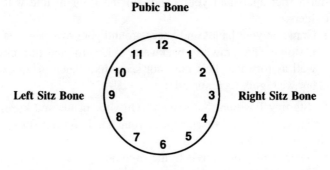

4. Starting Position: Same as 1. (Sit with your legs folded in front of you or with the soles of your feet touching in front of you.)

 • With your arms hanging by your sides, slowly slide your hands up the sides of your body and continue raising your hands and arms until your arms are extended overhead. Allow your focus to slowly move upward with your hands. Reverse the sequence to bring your arms back down. Repeat several times and observe what happens in your spine as your head and arms go up and down.

 • Take your arms up and down in the same manner, but this time move your head down as your arms move and move it up as your arms move down. This may feel strange, so do it as slowly as you need to. Again, observe what happens in your spine when you move your head and spine in this relationship.

Hands and Knees

If you have developed carpal tunnel syndrome (pressure on the median nerve at the point where it goes through the carpal tunnel of the wrist), this position may be painful. However, you can adjust the starting position by simply resting your forearms and/or chest on a chair or couch. If even that bothers you, skip the exercises in this position.

5. Starting Position: On your hands and knees with your knees about a foot apart and your hands on the floor in line with your shoulders.

- Crawl on your hands and knees around your exercise area. Take it slowly. Try crawling backward, sideward, and in a circle as well as forward. This may not seem like much of an exercise but we highly recommend it.

6. Starting Position: Same as 5. (On your hands and knees with your knees about a foot apart and your hands on the floor in line with your shoulders.)

- Gently shift your pelvis to the right and to the left a few times. Then add your head to this movement by looking over your right shoulder as you shift your pelvis to the right and over your left shoulder as you shift your pelvis to the left. Alternate slowly from side to side.

7. Starting Position: Same as 5. (On your hands and knees with your knees about a foot apart and your hands on the floor in line with your shoulders.)

- Keeping your hands in place on the floor, "push" into the floor with your hands and allow your torso to move back toward your heels. You may want to spread your knees farther apart to do this exercise. Once you're back as far as you can go (it's not necessary that your buttocks touch your heels), stay there for a while if you like. Most pregnant women find this a very comfortable position. When you are ready to return to the starting position, press into the floor with your lower legs (which are resting on the floor) and you will easily come back to your hands-and-knees.

8. Starting Position: Same as 5. (On your hands and knees with your knees about a foot apart and your hands on the floor in line with your shoulders.)

- Round your spine upward toward the ceiling like a cat. Imagine that you are draped over a huge ball. Return to the basic hands-and-knees position before you repeat.

Standing

9. Starting Position: Stand with your feet about shoulder width apart and your knees slightly bent.

- Slowly turn your head to the right and then back to the left. When you turn to the right, think about moving your head away from the left shoulder. When you turn to the left, think about moving your head away from the right shoulder. Do it several times. Only go as far as is comfortable. There should be no strain in your neck or shoulders.
- Slowly tilt your head up and down several times.
- Alternate tilting your head to the right and to the left. Think of your right ear moving toward your right shoulder as you tilt to the right and your left ear moving toward your left shoulder as you tilt to the left. Allow your shoulders to stay right where they are.
- Slowly circle your head in one direction and then the other. Repeat several times slowly. Observe what happens in the rest of your spine as you move only your head.

10. Starting Position: Same as 9. (Stand with your feet about shoulder width apart and your knees slightly bent.)

- Elbows bent, hands should be at shoulder level, palms facing outwards and to each side. Press your arms horizontally out to the sides, as if you were pressing two walls away from each other. With each press, bend and straighten your knees. In dancers' terms, do a small plié with each press.
- Press your arms in different directions. You can easily press them up, down, or directly in front of you. Experiment on your own. Just remember to pretend that you have walls to press apart, regardless of the direction you are pressing in.

11. Starting Position: Same as 9. (Stand with your feet about shoulder width apart and your knees slightly bent.)

- Curl your right toes under and then straighten them out again. Imagine that you are picking up a pencil with your toes. Do this several times and then try it with your left foot.

- Move your right foot outward, leaving your heel in place. Reverse directions and move it inward. Try both movements with your other foot.

12. Starting Position: Same as 9. (Stand with your feet about shoulder width apart and your knees slightly bent.)
- Stand in place and lift your legs alternately, trying to lift your knee as high as you easily can. This is one of those exercises where your belly will get in the way. Try this exercise starting with your feet parallel and then try it with your feet slightly turned out. Remember, no straining.

Recommended Reading

Prenatal Care

Eisenberg, Arlene; Murkoff, Heidi Eisenberg; and Eisenberg-Hathaway, Sandee, R.N. *What to Expect When You're Expecting.* New York: Workman Publishing, 1987.

Lesko, Wendy and Matthew. *The Maternity Sourcebook.* New York: Warner Books, 1984.

Simkin, Penny, et al. *Pregnancy, Childbirth and the Newborn.* Deephaven, MN: Meadowbrook, 1984.

Stoppard, Dr. Miriam. *Pregnancy and Birth Book.* New York: Ballantine, 1987.

Nutrition

Brewer, Tom. *Diet for Normal and High Risk Pregnancy.* New York: Simon and Schuster, 1983.

————. *What Every Pregnant Woman Should Know.* New York: Penguin, 1985.

Chubet, Carolyn T. *Feeding Your Baby.* Stamford, CT: Longmeadow, 1988.

Eden, Alvin N., M.D. *Dr. Eden's Healthy Kids.* New York: Signet, 1987.

Eisenberg, Arlene; Eisenberg, Heidi; Eisenberg-Hathaway, Sandee, R.N. *What to Eat When You're Expecting*. New York: Workman Publishing, 1986.

Fish, Helen; Fish, Ronald B.; and Golding, Lawrence A. *Starting Out Well*. Champaign, IL: Leisure Press, 1989.

The National Academy Press. *Nutrition During Pregnancy*. U.S. Dept. of Health, 1991.

Budgeting

Barker, Becky. *Answers: A Practical Survival Kit to Help You Organize Your Personal and Financial Matters*. New York: HarperCollins, 1991.

Crumbley, D. Lawrence, and Smith, L. Murphy. *Keys to Personal Financial Planning*. Hauppauge, NY: Barron, 1991.

Evans, Michael K. *How to Make Your Shrinking Salary Support You in Style*. New York: Random House, 1991.

Marshall Loeb's 1991 Money Guide. Boston: Little, Brown, 1990.

Quinn, Jane Bryant. *Making the Most of Your Money*. New York: Simon and Schuster, 1991.

Sprouse, Mary L. *Sprouse's Two Earner Money Book*. New York: Viking, 1991.

CHAPTER THREE

Class 3—Week 37

What's in This Chapter

The Payoff: Second Stage of Labor

After the Fact: Third and Fourth Stages

Lamaze Breathing: Pattern-paced

For the Coaches: Required Reading

Work Issues: Pregnant on the Job

Taking Care of Yourself: Things to Do and Lots of Them

Exercises

The Payoff: Second Stage of Labor

Let's begin with some confusion. Since there are four stages of labor, you may have thought that the last one is when your baby actually emerges. Plausible, but incorrect. Your baby is born at the conclusion of the second stage, and then other, much less exciting things happen in the third and fourth stages. The subject now is the second stage, the one you will have been waiting for all those months.

By the second stage your cervix will have dilated completely (about 10 cm) and you are able to push your baby out. You'll be tired from the first stage but you'll also be very excited about seeing your new baby and will probably have a renewed sense of energy.

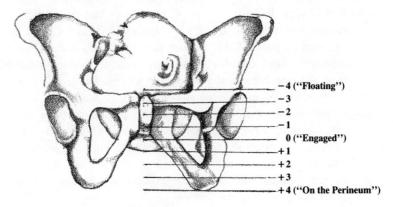

Pelvic Station

The second stage can last from 15 minutes to 3 hours or more. Your contractions last longer—between 50 and 70 seconds—and are closer together—2 1/2 to 4 minutes apart.

During this stage, your doctor may refer to your baby as being at a –4 station, 0 station, or +2 station. Translated, this number indicates how far your baby has descended in its journey from your uterus and through your vagina. It starts at the –5 station and is just about to emerge into the world (technically, is "on the perineum") at the +5 station. "Engaged" means that the baby has descended to the middle of the pelvis, or is at 0 station. The other stations denote whether the baby is above the middle of the pelvis or below the middle of the pelvis. This might seem—no, it is—a little confusing, but it's the standard medical jargon, and you'll want to know what your doctor is talking about. Just remember, the higher the positive number, the closer you are to delivering.

About Pushing

Pushing your baby through the birth canal is probably your biggest job. For some women, it's the most gratifying part of childbirth. The pain may not be as intense as it has been, and you will become more focused on getting the baby out, and less concerned with anything else going on.

The urge to push is an incredibly compelling, overpowering sensation that is very difficult to control. (If you've had an epidural, this sensation will not be as strong.) You'll want your doctor present when you start to push. If this is your first baby, you usually can start pushing without the doctor present because pushing takes longer with the first baby, and your doctor will have time to get to you. However, if you are having a home birth or have had other children, you should wait until the doctor is present to push. No need to start pushing any earlier than you have to! When the urge to push overtakes you, do the fast-paced breathing you will learn in this chapter (see page 77) and have your coach call your nurse by using the call button. Your coach or your coach's backup should stay by your side from this moment on.

On average, you can fit in approximately three pushes with each contraction. Your doctor will urge you not to rush, but to bear down gently, which will prevent you from tearing. You will want to hold your breath and bear down in synchrony with your uterus. By taking two deep breaths before bearing down, you will allow more oxygen to get to the fetus when the uterus is relaxed, and allow the contraction to build.

At some point, you may be asked to stop pushing for one of several reasons. Your doctor may sense that you are close to tearing your perineum. The second shoulder can be difficult to deliver, and your doctor may want to slow things at this point. Or your doctor may need time to suction the baby's head when it's delivered because you had meconium staining in your amniotic fluid. If your doctor wants to slow things down and asks you to stop pushing, immediately begin the pattern-paced breathing, which you will learn in this chapter.

Don't worry about having a bowel movement when you are pushing. At least you are pushing in the right direction! This happens all the time. Doctors are not miffed in the least if this happens, so you shouldn't give it a second thought. Focus on your pushing and nothing else.

Contractions are usually 3 to 4 minutes apart at this stage. Work with them one at a time. Push with the contraction, and then rest. If you rest between contractions, any way you can, you won't get so exhausted. Rest by using any relaxation techniques that work for you. Stretch your legs between contractions. Close your eyes and visualize a beautiful beach.

Be willing to change positions if you feel you need to. Women use all kinds of positions to push their babies out. Use whatever position makes you comfortable, but make sure you know what options are available and don't be afraid to improvise. Just keep in mind that squatting positions give maximum room for your baby to move through your pelvis and flat lying positions restrict oxygen flow and cause you to push against gravity. Try to avoid lying on your back.

Positions for Pushing

Familiarize yourself with these different positions and practice your simulated contractions with the positions you feel are most comfortable for you. Whether you are practicing or actually pushing during delivery, try to keep your shoulders rounded forward so that your spine is curved in the shape of a C, regardless of the position you are in.

Squatting: Get a kitchen or dining-room chair, and, in a crouching position, feet flat on the floor and facing the chair, hold on to the chair and tuck your bottom under. You can also do this with your coach and hold on to his or her legs for support.

Ballet position: The ballet position is another "squatting" position, but use your coach for support instead of a chair. Have your coach sit in a chair and squat between your coach's legs, again feet flat on the floor and arms hanging on either side of the coach's legs. In the ballet position you face away from your coach.

Semireclining position: This position needs the help of your coach and your nurse. Lying on the bed, elevate your back with enough pillows so that you are halfway between sitting up and lying down. Bend your knees and place one foot against your coach's body and the other foot against your nurse's body. They will hold your legs to stabilize them as you push.

Toilet pushing: Sitting on the toilet is a natural place to push. Some women find this position so comfortable for pushing that they don't want to move even when it's time for the baby to emerge. This makes it tough.

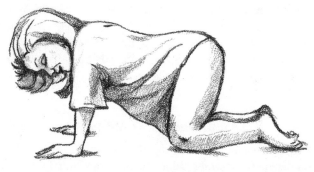

Hands and knees: Pushing when you are on your hands and knees will help rotate the positions of the baby, reduce backache, and allow you plenty of free movement. It's a good position to have in your repertoire. Just be sure you have a soft enough surface so your knees have some protection.

On your back: Lie on your back and pull your legs back with your hands. Place your hands on the back of your knees. Raise your head, pull back your legs, and push.

Taylor sit: Sit with your legs in front of you, knees bent and soles of your feet together. A variation of this position is to sit with pillows behind you and hold on to the backs of your knees. (Your feet are not together in this variation.)

Lithotomy: This position may be necessary for forceps or vacuum deliveries. You will be asked to lie on your back with your legs raised in the stirrups and with your hips on the edge of the table.

Birthing chairs: Many facilities now have birthing chairs. It has been reported that using one can reduce back pain, increase spontaneous birth (no intervention), and shorten the active stage. When you use one, you are in an upright position, which also facilitates second-stage labor. If your facility has one, you will be instructed how to use it when you take your preliminary tour of the facility.

The Birth

As we said, the second stage also includes the actual birth of your baby. The second stage is officially over when you have pushed your baby completely out. However, there's a lot more going on besides pushing.

Tearing

If you're going to tear, this is when it will happen, usually when the head or the second shoulder is delivered. But there's nothing to fear.

Perineal tears can be large or small, and are described by degrees from 1 to 4. A first-degree tear is the smallest; fourth-degree is the largest, and needs the most repair. Many women feel terrible if they tear. Some want to have a "perfect" delivery, and a tear does not fit in that category. But the reasons for tears are out of your control, so don't blame yourself. Perineal tears commonly occur if babies are big or if they come out fast. Those are both good situations, so the tear might be looked on as a small price to pay. (And there's nothing much you can do about it, anyway.)

The Delivery

When you are pushing, you will feel a stretching sensation. That's when the baby's head is emerging. At this point, they will let you look in the mirror and see the baby's head. If you have your eyes closed, open them so that you can see the baby. Often this will give you a renewed burst of strength.

You don't have to wait until they cut the cord to have your first contact with your child. Ask if you can touch the baby's head as it emerges. It will feel soft and squishy. Some doctors will also let you lift the baby out yourself.

Suctioning the Baby

Your baby's mouth and nose will be suctioned with a long, thin suction tube or a nasal bulb aspirator as soon as his or her head is delivered. You may be asked to do your pattern-paced breathing a few times once the head is delivered, so the doctor has time to suction the mouth and nose before the rest of the baby is delivered.

For the record, the actual birth of the baby marks the transition between the second and third stages of delivery.

After the Fact: Third and Fourth Stages

The third stage begins with the birth of the baby and ends with the delivery of the placenta. Repairs for tears or episiotomy will also be done now. The third stage can take from ten to thirty minutes, but you probably won't care how long it takes. You'll be so wrapped up in your new baby that you won't care what is going on around you. But here's what does happen during this stage.

Cutting the Cord

Most hospitals allow the coach the option of cutting the umbilical cord. Your doctor is more concerned about when the cord is cut rather than who cuts it. Old theory stated that the cord should be cut after it stopped pulsating. However, the new theory is that the baby gets too much blood and becomes jaundiced if the wait to cut the cord is too long.

So, if your coach wants to cut the cord, he or she should speak up as soon as the baby is delivered. This option might have been discussed beforehand with your doctor. Some coaches will respectfully pass, and that is their privilege.

Determining the Sex

Do it yourselves. This may seem like a minor point but it's much nicer for the coach to be the one to tell you the sex of your baby (if you don't already know).

Placenta Delivery

Most women don't mind this event, but some women are so exhausted they literally cannot do any more. A friend in this condition told her doctor in no uncertain terms that if she wanted the placenta, she was going to have to go in there and get it herself! This is an exaggeration, and, usually, the placenta is pushed out by the uterine contractions and you don't have to do any work.

The placenta is normally delivered when the uterus contracts and pulls away from the placenta. (You may need to do your pattern-paced breathing as the uterus contracts.) The placenta is usually delivered in one piece. Many people like to see it, so don't be afraid to ask.

Occasionally, there is trouble delivering the placenta, and the doctor may have to go up inside and pull the placenta off the uterine wall. If this procedure becomes too uncomfortable, they may take you into the delivery room and give you a quick general anesthesia. You will be brought right back to your husband and baby after the procedure. It is very important to remove all the placenta; otherwise, you can hemorrhage.

Repair

If you have a tear or an episiotomy (a surgical incision) that needs repair, they will sew it up now. A first-degree tear may not need any sutures, but a fourth-degree tear (from the vagina down to the rectum) definitely needs to be stitched.

Time Alone

The coach should get everyone calm and quiet and comfortable after the birth, and negotiate for some time alone together with the new baby. Try to avoid separation. This is the first moment that you are joined as a family unit, and it should be very special. Most hospital staffs are aware of the importance of this quiet time, and will honor it. You will probably want to try to nurse at this time, if you are planning on doing so. It's a very important time for bonding.

After-Delivery Care for the Baby

You've delivered your baby, and now all you want to do is hold your child. While you're holding the baby, they will place an ID bracelet on your baby's ankle or wrist, do an overall check, counting fingers and toes, etc., and do an Apgar Score. However, one to two hours after the baby is born, the nurse or doctor will take your baby away for a routine examination in the labor room. The same routine is followed in a birthing center or by your midwife if you have a home birth. We explain the major procedures of after care below.

Apgar score: This score is done twice, the first time one minute after the baby is born and the second five minutes after the baby is born. To call it a test is a little misleading, because it is actually just an observation of the baby's color and other basic reactions like breathing and crying. However, it is like a test in that the observations are scored. Unfortunately, the description of the scores can be alarming. A score of 7 to 10 is considered normal, 4 to 6 mild to moderate depression, 0 to 3 severe depression. The score usually improves on the second test, although a low score is not necessarily anything to become alarmed at.

Eye drops or ointment: This varies from hospital to hospital, and is often delayed until two hours after birth so that parents and babies can see each other clearly without having the drops or ointment impair the baby's vision. Some facilities administer silver nitrate drops, and others administer erythromycin ointment. Silver nitrate tends to irritate the baby's eyes more. Both have the same purpose: protection against venereal disease.

Washing: The nurse will wash the baby with mild soap and warm water.

Weighing: The nurse will weigh the baby and record its birth weight.

Measuring: The nurse will record the baby's length.

PKU test: This is a blood test that determines how the baby is processing protein. Blood is usually drawn from the baby's heel. This test is usually done 48 hours after birth.

Vitamin K shot: Helps in clotting, and it is especially helpful for breastfeeding moms who do not pass along a lot of Vitamin K through their breast milk.

Vital signs: The baby's blood pressure, heart rate, temperature, and respirations are recorded.

The fourth stage begins after the placenta has been delivered, and lasts from one to two hours following the birth of the baby until the mother's condition is stabilized. Most women are still very excited at this stage, and it takes time to calm down. Your coach can be with you.

During this period, your legs might shake uncontrollably from the strain of labor. A warm blanket can help relieve the shaking. You may also experience "afterpains" which is actually the uterus contracting. These pains will subside in a few hours. The key point here is: it's over. You're not pregnant any longer!

Lamaze Breathing: Pattern-paced

The third type of breathing is called *pattern-paced breathing*. It is normally used during the second stage of labor when you are ready to push, and can be used to carry you through the peak of a contraction. However, when you are practicing this pattern, obviously you don't want to push. So, when you're practicing, the instructions will be to hold your breath for a certain number of counts instead of pushing.

Like moderate-paced breathing, your respiration rate for pattern-paced breathing should not exceed 24 breaths per minute. Your inhalations should be light and shallow. The exhalations should be short and quick, like blowing out a candle.

You've had so much breathing practice by this point you'll pick this technique up very quickly. We'll give you two versions to try.

Version 1. One-breath pattern

1. Inhale slowly and easily.
2. Exhale with a "ha" or "whroo" (whichever you prefer).
3. Inhale slowly and easily.
4. Bear down (hold your breath for 6 counts).

Version 2. Two-breath pattern

1. Inhale slowly and easily.
2. Exhale with a "ha" or "whroo."
3. Inhale slowly and easily.
4. Exhale with a "ha" or "whroo."
5. Inhale slowly and easily.
6. Bear down (hold your breath for 6 counts).

The following breathing practice will give you a chance to practice the two versions of pattern-paced breathing. Take it slowly the first couple of times through. You'll probably find you like one version better than the other.

As you become more comfortable with all of these breathing exercises, try to focus on the number of breaths you take, and make sure your respiration rate is not getting too high. The more you practice breathing slowly, the more automatic it will become, which is what you will need in labor. When you are in true labor, it will be tough to focus on the number of breaths that you take per minute.

Your coach can also try something new in this practice session. To indicate the intensity of the contractions, he or she can squeeze your hand when the contraction begins to intensify, and squeeze it again when it begins to subside. As you practice, remind your coach to vary the pace and peak of the contractions.

1. Indicate to your partner that the contraction is beginning. Begin timing the contraction.

   Contraction begins. Take a deep cleansing breath.

2. Squeeze your partner's hand to indicate contraction is increasing.

   Begin the pattern-paced breathing. Inhale and exhale with ha, inhale and hold 1–2–3–4–5–6 (or inhale and exhale

**with ha, inhale and exhale with ha, inhale and hold
1–2–3–4–5–6).**

3. **Contraction ends. Take a deep cleansing breath.**

Repeat as many times as needed to get the hang of it.

For the Coaches: Required Reading

To be honest, many coaches are not enthusiastic about attending childbirth classes. Nor do they want to read books. They think they can just show up when the time comes and act cool. It doesn't work that way. These are the coaches who get weak knees the minute they walk into the hospital or birth center, panic with the first contraction, faint at the sight of blood, and are of no help to their partners. If you as a coach find yourself slipping into an easygoing attitude, we urge you to reconsider. In order to be *beneficially* cool under fire, you have to be prepared. Remember, you have the easiest part of the job, by definition. You should be prepared to do it right.

As the coach, you are an integral part of the Lamaze method, sometimes even referred to as "verbal anesthesia." Not an elegant phrase, but you get the point: a solid, dependable coach really helps at the moment of truth. And although you, the coach, may be as inexperienced as the woman you are assisting, you can easily learn the Lamaze fundamentals. The main point for you to know is that you are there to help your partner, whatever that means, and provide all the moral support she needs. *She* can panic; you can't.

At the very least, you will need to be prepared to stay with her, or be sure that someone else is there with her, through the entire labor. Of course, you will be prepared to assist in getting through the contractions, but you will also find yourself helping the expectant mother relax, acting as a liaison with the hospital staff, and perhaps taking absolute control of the whole process should your partner lose it, which is not that unusual. Here are a few general suggestions to keep in mind for any and all eventualities.

Encourage Her

It is your job as coach to encourage your partner to go on. Give her special looks, squeeze her hand, and offer many, many words of encouragement: "You're all right, loosen your shoulders, open your body, let the baby out, give way, you're doing fine." Have faith in her ability to go on, even if she doesn't.

Keep Her Comfortable

The job that may keep you the busiest is keeping your partner comfortable. Pay attention and use your intuition. Look at her, see what she needs, then do it! One woman we know, Maggie, actually used her midwife as her coach. Maggie felt great when, in heavy labor, she could bite on her coach-midwife's sleeve. But when it became too hot in the labor room, the coach decided to roll up her sleeves—and Maggie, otherwise engaged, failed to notice. So when the next contraction began, Maggie started to bite down anyway. A close call! Her coach immediately rolled down her sleeves and Maggie continued chewing. For the coach, anything goes.

- Set the mood. Keep the atmosphere light with your tone of voice. Play some of your partner's favorite tapes as background music.
- Keep her hydrated. Offer water, juice, and ice chips, and make sure she takes liquids in some form.
- Keep her cool. Place a cold cloth on her forehead. Sponge off her entire body with a cold cloth. Fan if necessary. Better yet, be sure an electric fan is available.
- Be her masseuse or masseur. Try different techniques. One massage technique is to begin by using a light touch to relieve surface tension. Use long, flowing, downward strokes to generally relax muscles. Use thumb pressure at each side of the spine to relieve pressure on the sacrum and coccyx. To specifically relieve back pain, use firm pressure on the lower back. Remember the tennis-ball technique. Whatever technique you try, be sure to use talcum powder, lotion, or oil to reduce skin friction.

We should mention here that some women do not like to be touched during contractions—and this eccentricity might not emerge until that very moment. They might love massages otherwise. As the coach, do not argue. Definitely do not say, "But you—"

Go with the flow. Even touching the bed can be irritating, so be extra-sensitive to your partner's needs. As mentioned before, one woman we know stood in the shower during her worst contractions, and wanted no one to touch her, including her husband the coach. Fine. These are, after all, what we call extenuating circumstances.

Be Her Advocate

It will be your job to interact with the birth attendants. The nurses will depend on you to give them feedback on your partner's specific needs and problems, such as not wanting to be touched.

But you may also have to interact with the nurses or other attendants in more assertive ways. For example, it's common (too common) for the physician or other caregiver to start doing a procedure without discussing it with the coach or your partner. Your partner may be in no position to stand up for herself and ask what's going on. But this is what she has you for. One coach we know really had to get pushy. Just when his wife was ready for the final push, everyone in the room started shouting orders. So he yelled, "Shut up!" This stunned everyone, but did accomplish the main goal. His wife was able to focus and push the baby out.

Prepare for the Unexpected

Be prepared for the unexpected during labor and delivery. The unexpected includes complications in the delivery as well as in your wife's behavior. These latter surprises are now the subject. Giving birth generates a full range of contrasting feelings and reactions: excitement, fear, relief, anger, panic, calm, weariness, strength, detachment, self-doubt, confidence. As the coach, you need to be able to handle all of them. Many laboring women have called their loved ones some not-so-loving names during this time. They might even become temporarily aggressive: one coach told us that his wife, who normally loves to have her back rubbed, swung her arm back and hit him when he started a massage. No problem. He got the message.

Helping with Contractions

Your main job as coach will be to work through each contraction with your partner. It will be your job to:

- Help her take one contraction at a time.
- Encourage mobility and variety of positions: shower, toilet, standing, walking, squatting, all fours, leaning.
- Pace her and follow the rhythm of her contractions, keeping eye contact, nodding your head in time with her breathing, matching her breathing with your own, talking in a soothing monotone, stroking her in rhythm with each breath.
- Focus on her breathing. Knowing what pattern of breathing will be most helpful will make you feel much more in control and can help your partner's discomfort.
- Realize when the "downhill" side of each contraction has begun, and help her slow down.

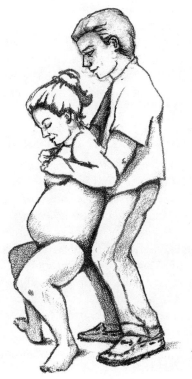

- Talk her through the strong contractions in a steady, calm monotone, such as: "Great, terrific, open up even more, each breath—all the way down, you're doing fine, keep with it, beautiful, let it go now, all the way through, easy, fine, relax even more, super!"
- Offer visualization suggestions to help her through each contraction. Convey calm, peace, floating, stillness, softness, heaviness, flowing.
- Give her physical support. Rock her in your arms in rhythm with her breathing. Let her squeeze you or pound rhythmically on you or just cling to you. Remind her to keep her buttocks loose.

Know When and How to Take Control

Some women in labor feel like they just cannot go on anymore, and suddenly find themselves out of control. Their contractions are a lot more intense, they get discouraged and possibly irrational, and then they lose the focus on their breathing. Once they lose control, the contractions will feel much worse, and it is difficult to get back into the rhythm. Let her give in to her body, and go with the contractions rather than fight them. Coach, this is when you will be needed the most. This is your shining hour!

It's your job to get things back to normal—well, not normal, but acceptable—any way you can. You must take control. Use your voice, your touch, and eye contact to make your partner focus and do what you tell her to do. Offer positive suggestions to replace unproductive behavior. Replace screaming with low-pitched sound; replace flailing motions with rocking motions. Get in her face and breathe with her and keep her on track any way you can.

Work Issues: Pregnant on the Job

Certain conditions such as fatigue and backache come with the territory of being pregnant. Some women make it through their pregnancies without being bothered by these or other complaints to be enumerated shortly, but most pregnant women will experience them at one time or another, whether at home or at work. Obviously, it's easier to take countermeasures at home: lie down and take a long nap. It's not so easy at work. Nevertheless, pregnancy is usually no reason for any drastic change in your attendance or performance record at work, should you choose to continue working until late in your term. There are ways to cope.

However, if you are simply unable to work because of a pregnancy-related condition, you are entitled to "sick days" or, should it come to it, disability leave, just like other employees. Many pregnant women are uncomfortable taking the sick days they are entitled to. Don't be too hard on yourself. If you are forced to cut back or take extra time off for legitimate health reasons, don't feel guilty. If you weren't pregnant, you would take vacation days or sick days without the blink of an eye. Why make yourself feel guilty over something that you are entitled to? Besides, you won't impress anyone by showing up unable to do your job.

Now let's take a look at some of the common conditions of pregnancy that may adversely affect you, and offer suggestions how to cope with them at work.

Morning Sickness

The cause of morning sickness is unclear, but blame is usually placed on the increased level of the HCG hormone. The term itself is unclear, or at least inaccurate, because women may experience morning sickness at 4 P.M.. or 12 midnight. The symptoms are clear enough, however: nausea and vomiting. If you are fated to have trouble with morning sickness—and two-thirds of pregnant women do—it will probably "strike" between the second and sixth weeks of pregnancy, and then end at the twelfth week or thereabouts. However, some women have to deal with it throughout their pregnancy.

Remedies for morning sickness come in and out of fashion. Gingersnaps, which supposedly reduce the acidity in the stomach, have come into fashion lately. Eating dry carbohydrates before you even get out of bed in the morning, for frequent snacks, and whenever your stomach feels upset seems to help, as well. Eat frequent, small meals as often as every couple of hours, and avoid smelly, spicy, or greasy foods. Some women have found that vitamin B-6 helps with morning sickness. Others swear by herbal teas. (Check with your doctor/midwife before drinking any "unusual" herbal teas.) If iced water with exactly seven cubes works for you, we say, "Go for it!" However, check with your doctor before taking any bizarre "remedies" you may have heard about through the grapevine. And if you are truly incapacitated by morning sickness, your doctor may recommend medication, such as Emetrol.

Lack of Energy

Fatigue affects almost all pregnant women at some point. The reasons are obvious enough: your body is very busy, copious amounts of hormones are causing tremendous physical and emotional changes, your sleep is probably disrupted by frequent urination at night. You will probably experience the greatest fatigue in the first three months. Then you'll reenergize; but late in pregnancy, carrying around all this extra weight, you'll tire easily again.

Rest is the only sure treatment. Make sure you get to bed early. If you feel the urination factor at night is especially disruptive, cut down on your intake of liquids in the evening. Take a nap when you get home from work, if possible, or spend ten minutes doing your relaxation exercises. If you have a private office, you just might be able to squeeze in a quick nap. Some women find that if they get out of the office at lunchtime and take a brisk walk they are energized for the afternoon.

If your work and schedule are flexible, make the most of that flexibility. If you drag in the mornings, take care of the easier work then. Save the tough stuff for when you're sharper. Or vice versa. Perhaps your hours can be changed to take advantage of when you're at your best. A teacher we know was used to staying after school to do her grading and class preparations. When she became pregnant, she was out of gas by three o'clock. She discovered that if she took her work home instead of staying at school, she could take a nap, do her paperwork, and still have time to help her husband with dinner. We can't guarantee that any of these suggestions will work for you, but if you find yourself struggling, you'll also find yourself trying various tactics to figure out what works best.

Backaches

As we discussed in Chapter One, your lower back will bother you on and off throughout your pregnancy. You are instinctively making postural compensations—such as tilting backward with your upper body—for your larger size and weight. A loosening of the joints also contributes to strain on the muscles and ligaments of the lower back and legs.

Exercise is often recommended for this low backache. However, if you're at work, it will probably be totally inappropriate to pause in your duties and do pelvic-tilt exercises. If it's not inappropriate— if you're the boss—by all means do those exercises! Otherwise, you may obtain some relief simply by moving your back around as you sit or stand. Rock your pelvis forward and back. Move your pelvis around as if you are drawing a circle with your tailbone. If you're sitting, shift from one buttock to the other, back and forth, back and forth. These movements can be so inconspicuous that no one will notice. Besides, people in general shift around in their chairs and while they're standing because it's uncomfortable to sit or stand in one position for any extended time. You'll just be making your shifting worthwhile.

Try to wear low-heeled shoes with cushioned soles. High heels put more stress on your lower back. One note of caution: If you normally wear high heels, come down to low heels gradually. Your calf muscles may be too tight from wearing high-heeled shoes to go to the other extreme too suddenly.

If you sit at a desk all day and your feet don't touch the ground, place a fat phone book or two under your desk so your feet have support. Occasionally you might let your toes rest on the phone book, with your heels touching the floor. This may seem like a pretty trivial suggestion, but it will definitely decrease the stress on your lower back.

Placing a firm pillow at the small of your back when you are sitting in any kind of chair supports your back and relieves some of the strain. At night, sleep on your side and place a pillow between your legs. Some women have to place a small pillow under their stomachs in this position, so they don't feel "weighed over."

Emotional Swings

As explained in Chapter One, your changing hormones can cause extreme emotional swings, which can occur anywhere, at any time. However, your emotional swings at work can be more of a hindrance than those at home. The most common, potentially embarrassing swing will be some kind of out-of-character overreaction. You say something you would normally never say, and immediately regret it. Or you may flush with inappropriate anger or sadness. And you'll be caught off guard by these emotions.

The best advice we can offer is that you make a habit of taking a deep breath or two before you react to anything. Sometimes that's all that's needed to let your hormones know that you, not they, are still in control. But if you do react in some off-the-wall manner, don't pretend that nothing happened. Make things right. Apologize for undue anger or misspoken words. If you made a bad decision, change it. Don't be concerned that people will be condescending or overly sympathetic just because "she's pregnant." You *are* pregnant. That's the fact and everyone knows it (we presume).

Low Blood Sugar

Your body's need for carbohydrates increases tremendously during pregnancy. It turns these raw materials into the simple sugar glucose, which provides you and your fetus with energy. This constant demand for energy can also cause sudden drops in blood sugar, often accompanied by sudden irritability. To avoid this, you may need to snack more often. Eating six small meals a day helps your body metabolize your food better.

Unless you are an assembly-line worker, you can probably arrange a few small meals or snacks during work hours. If your office doesn't have a refrigerator or microwave, keep crackers, granola bars, trail mix, etc., in your office. If you're out of your office for extended periods of time, keep a few packages in your purse or briefcase. Just remember that your snack should provide nutrition as well as ease your hunger.

Edema

The requirements of many jobs contribute to or aggravate edema. If you have edema or want to avoid it, try to avoid standing or sitting for long periods. If you have to sit, avoid crossing your legs; sit with your feet elevated at whatever angle is comfortable and appropriate. Our friend the schoolteacher needed to elevate her legs when seated at her desk, but the first time she tried it in her classroom all of her students followed suit. Imagine twenty third-graders with their feet on their desks! She quickly had to explain why she could do it and they could not.

If you have to stand upright in your job, try to keep moving. Walking will do wonders for your circulation, but even just shifting your weight back and forth from one foot to another is helpful. Avoid standing still at all costs.

The way you dress can help, too. Wear support stockings—and be sure to put them on before you get out of bed in the morning, before the blood has any chance to pool. Avoid any type of tight clothing, especially at the waist and ankles.

Taking Care of Yourself:
Things to Do and Lots of Them

It would be nice if all you had to do to prepare for the birth of your child was to do your breathing and relaxation exercises. Unfortunately, that's not the case. Weeks before you deliver, at minimum, you need to have selected a hospital or birth center (if you're not having the baby at home), preregistered at the facility, chosen a pediatrician, packed your bag for the hospital, and stocked up on baby supplies. Buying Q-Tips is not so difficult, but if you've never had a child before, how do you find a hospital or pediatrician or family practitioner? You know you need to take your toothbrush to the hospital, but what else will you need? Here are the ABCs.

First Things First: Where Are You Going to Have this Baby?

You probably know where you want to have your baby, but just in case you don't, we'll briefly go over your options. The most common and traditional location is in a hospital. However, more and more women are choosing birthing centers, which can either be part of a hospital or free-standing, or they are opting for home births. Where you choose will partly depend on your medical condition during pregnancy and, occasionally, during labor.

Hospitals are the most common choice because they are the safest facilities. They are staffed with medical personnel and equipped with the lastest technology, making some mothers feel more confident and comfortable. Insurance usually covers deliveries in hospitals.

Birth centers are staffed by nurses and nurse-midwives. They tend to rely on less medical intervention, although they have all the latest equipment too. They also support natural childbirth and bonding, are very open to family and friends, and are slightly less expensive than hospitals. The average stay in a birthing center is also shorter. In fact, they normally send you home about twelve hours after you deliver. Insurance usually covers birthing centers also, but you should check your individual policy.

The advantages of a delivery at home are obvious and not to be underestimated: familiarity, the best possible environment for bonding, conditions totally subject to your own control, and the least expensive option. The one major concern with home births is that, should a serious complication arise, you're in the wrong place for quick medical intervention.

Preregister at a Hospital or Birthing Center

This is something you *must* do. In order to convince you of this, let's sketch this scenario, which is not hypothetical. It happens. You show up at the hospital for the first time having bona fide contractions. No false labor, this. But instead of being able to proceed straight to the maternity floor, you are asked to fill out all the necessary insurance information and hoopla. Not the kind of thing you enjoy doing under normal circumstances, and you certainly don't want to be bothered with it while you're trying to deliver a baby. If you're lucky, you and your coach will be on your way to the maternity floor within 45 to 60 minutes of filling out the forms and waiting for clerical approval. This can be a very long time if you are having contractions. Or this might happen: You're zipped up to the maternity floor, directed to a labor room, and left with a nurse. Your coach stays behind and fills out all the forms. At this point, you want your coach by your side all the time. Take our word for it.

No one should have to start her delivery under circumstances even remotely similar to these. We highly recommend preregistration. It's so easy. Many hospitals and birthing centers even offer preregistration by mail. Normally, doctors will give you a card that you can fill out with your name, address, and due date. They in turn will give this information to the admissions people at the facility of your choice. Once they receive your card, they send out a packet of information, which will contain insurance information, an anesthesiologist questionnaire form, and emergency numbers. When you return your completed packet to the admitting office, they verify all the insurance information. You are now painlessly preregistered and ready to go.

If your doctor does not offer to assist you with preregistration, you will need to go to the admitting office at your hospital or birthing center and fill out all the forms. Not quite as easy as doing it by mail, but better than the alternative.

Sign a Consent Form

This is usually the last thing you think about, if you think about it at all, but it could be one of the first things you need. A consent form gives the hospital and doctor permission to do whatever is necessary during your delivery. Sometimes you are able to sign the form at your doctor's office. Usually, you will sign it on one of your last office visits. Your doctor's office then sends the consent form over to the hospital. However, many hospitals control the consent forms and you might have to go to the hospital to sign it. Ask your doctor about this, in case you do have to make a personal appearance at the hospital.

Interview Pediatricians or Family Practitioners

You need to have a doctor on hand to check out your new baby medically. If you haven't found one before you go to the hospital, or if for some reason yours is not available, the pediatric resident will serve as your pediatrician.

To find a pediatrician or family practitioner for your baby, ask for recommendations from your doctor and other parents you know. Then take the time to personally consider these recommendations. A call to the doctor's office will answer many routine questions, such as the cost of office visits and the schedule for office hours. But to find out if this is the right doctor for your child, you'll need to interview him or her in person. Make the time to do it.

In your interview with a pediatrician, be sure to ask questions that will give you an idea of this person's philosophy of child care and style of practice. Weigh that information with practical considerations, such as the location of the office, the office hours, and the fees. With all that information, the decision won't be difficult to make.

The following are common questions that people ask when interviewing pediatricians. You probably have many of your own. To ensure that all your questions are answered, take your list of questions with you and do not hesitate to consult it.

Questions for the Doctor:
- Is there a cost for the initial consultation?
- Is the doctor supportive of breastfeeding? At what age are solids introduced?
- What are her/his views on circumcision?
- What are her/his attitudes about working mothers?
- Does the doctor have a pediatric nurse-practitioner?
- What are her/his feelings about telephone calls for minor problems?
- Does the doctor have staff privileges at your hospital? This is necessary for the baby's discharge. You will need to contact a pediatrician who practices at your hospital to discharge your baby.
- How large is the practice?
- Do appointments have to be made far in advance?
- If it is a group practice, how does the "on call" schedule work?
- Do you see the same doctor each visit?

- How does the fee schedule work? Is there a package plan for newborns?
- How often is a baby seen in the office? Does the doctor make home visits? Is there an extra charge for home visits?
- If you are planning to use the Early Discharge Program be sure to inform your pediatrician.

Questions to Answer for Yourself:
- Where is the office located? It is preferable for the office to be close to your home.
- Do you feel comfortable just sitting and talking with the doctor?
- Are the fees affordable for you?
- Does the doctor make you feel that he or she has all the time in the world for you and your baby?
- How do the staff and doctors interact with their patients?
- Are there toys in the waiting room?
- Do the little patients seem to be petrified or are they oblivious and playing?
- Does the doctor explain everything (medical terms) to you so that you can understand?

Pack Your Bags

You don't want to be running around at the last minute trying to find camera film and clean underwear to take to the hospital. Give yourself a break and pack your bags at least one month before your due date.

We say bags—plural—because the list of what you need to take to the hospital or birthing center is long. You'll even need the same collection of items at home. So pack a bag even if you're having a home birth and in case it doesn't turn out that way at the last minute. You might want to organize everything into a couple of bags—perhaps one for items needed during labor and delivery, and one for everything else. You probably don't need your baby's going-home outfit in with the tennis balls for your back massage. We'll just provide the list. You organize and pack it any way you want to.

Women often refer to one of their hospital bags as their Lamaze bag. In the sixties, Lamaze instructors put together a list of what to take to the hospital, and now "Lamaze bag" is the generic term for the bag that contains everything you need during labor and delivery. The list has changed through the years, improved and refined by suggestions from mothers and coaches. You may want to substitute or add some items. Just make sure you have the essentials. And make certain that you pack early.

For Labor and Delivery

- Cornstarch or talcum powder—for massages. You will get sticky and sweaty, so we recommend cornstarch because it's easier for the coach to rub you with something that will absorb moisture. Cornstarch also has no odor.
- Vaseline/Chapstick. Your lips get dry.
- Focus object—something you like, perhaps, but mainly something that will do the job, as discussed in Chapter One.
- Socks—for cold feet.
- Tennis balls—for back massage.
- Hard-sour candy/lollipop: sweet candy is nauseating.
- Phone/address book for calls after delivery.
- Camera and lots of film.
- Hairbrush, ribbons, elastics for long hair.
- Change for parking meters in case you cannot park in the garage (you never know how long you are going to be).
- Cotton hat for baby after birth. Put on baby immediately after delivery.
- Tape recorder, battery operated, for music. Favorite tapes.
- Wine or champagne for after-delivery, if you so desire, and, in the case of vaginal deliveries, anything you would like for food.
- Paper lunch bags for hyperventilating.

For the Mother

- Two nightgowns (nursing nighties)
- Slippers
- Robe
- Two nursing bras (buy them one size larger than your pregnancy bras).

- Toilet articles
- Breast pump
- Clothes to wear home. Take clothes that fit you late in your pregnancy. The top should be something that you can easily breastfeed in.

For the Coach

- Comfortable clothes—Some coaches go straight from work to the hospital.
- Comfortable, cushioned shoes—You'll be on your feet a long time.
- Favorite snacks
- Swimsuit, for use in the shower

For Your Baby

- Car seat. It's the law in most states. Many hospitals won't allow you to leave the hospital with your baby unless you have a car seat.
- Padding for the car seat. Most car seats are too big for newborns and need padding so your baby fits snugly in it. Most children's stores sell padding designed for this purpose.
- Going-home outfit. Include a hat for warmth.
- Two receiving blankets.

Stocking Up at Home

Once you return home, there are certain items that you won't be able to get along without. If you don't want to send someone to the store the moment you return home and every fifteen minutes thereafter, take the list below to your local drugstore or supermarket and purchase everything on it, in the recommended quantities.

- Nasal bulb aspirator for mucus
- Baby nail clippers
- Three large boxes of stick-on sanitary napkins
- Rectal thermometer or tape thermometer
- Bottle of isopropyl alcohol as umbilical-cord cleanser

- Witch hazel or Tucks—two bottles, or two of these
- Cotton swabs
- Cotton balls
- Baby wipes
- Cornstarch: instead of baby powder
- Mobile for over crib: black/white and red are recommended
- Stroller

For Breastfeeding Mothers

- Lanolin/colostrum for nipples
- Breast pads: three boxes
- Nursing bras: three
- Nuk pacifiers: three

For Bottle-feeding Mothers

- Bottles
- Nipples
- Formula (1 case—only if bottle feeding)

Rent a Childbirth Video

When you take a formal childbirth class, the teacher usually shows you a film of an actual birth. As they say, a picture is worth a thousand words. If you are not attending a formal childbirth class, arrange for you and your coach to see a film. We recommend two: *A Child Is Born* from Time-Life Video, and *Childbirth Preparation Program* by the American College of Obstetricians and Gynecologists. You can rent these videos from many video stores and can check them out from most libraries. If you can't find either of them, contact your local hospital or your doctor.

Exercises

Some of these exercises are extensions of the exercises in Chapter Two, others are brand-new. Try them and see which ones you like and want to make part of your exercise program.

Sitting

1. Starting Position: Sit with your legs folded in front of you or with the soles of your feet touching in front of you.
- Shift your rib cage forward and backward several times.
- Shift your rib cage from left to right like a typewriter carriage.
- Draw an imaginary circle with your rib cage, starting small and gradually increasing the size of the circle the more times you draw it. Reverse directions.

2. Starting Position: Same as 1. (Sit with your legs folded in front of you or with the soles of your feet touching in front of you.)
- Rock left and right, from one sitz bone to the other as you did in Chapter Two. As you shift to the right, allow your upper body to twist gently to the right also. Twist far enough so that your left hip comes off the floor. Allow your hands to follow. Your right hand will touch the floor on your right side, followed by your left hand. Try it. It sounds more complicated than it is.
- Rock from left to right as in the exercise above but "cartwheel" your arms over as you shift and twist from side to side.
- Rock from left to right as in the exercise above but reach with your left arm to the right as you shift and twist to the right (allow your right hand to rest on the floor and catch some of your weight). Reach to the left with your right arm as you shift to the left and use your left hand for balance.

3. Starting Position: Sit with your legs in a wide V shape, with your knees bent and your feet flat on the floor.
- Move your right foot to meet your left foot and then return it to the beginning "bent" V position. Try this several times, alternating legs.
- Include your arms as you move your feet this time. Start with your legs in a V and your arms extended in a V in front of you as well. As you move your right leg to meet your left leg, move your right arm to your left arm. As you open your right leg to return to the V, open your right arm. Alternate sides.

4. Starting Position: Sit in a V with your legs extended.
- With your legs very loose, rotate your legs inward and outward.

5. Starting Position: Same as 4. (Sit in a V with your legs extended.)

- Slide your right foot in toward your body and then slide it out again. Alternate legs.
- Slide your right foot in toward your body and slide it out again, but this time slide it out next to your left leg. Slide your right foot in again and extend it again, returning to the original V position. Alternate legs.
- Add some arms movements to the above exercise. As you slide your right foot in toward your body, bend your elbow so that your hand comes close or touches your right shoulder. As you slide your right foot out parallel to your left leg, extend your right arm. In other words, let your arms copy your legs.

6. Starting position: Sit with your legs extended straight in front of you.

- Bend your feet and knees at the same time, then straighten them. Think about moving your knees and your toes to the ceiling as you flex, and back toward the floor as you extend. After you have that down, "pedal" alternately.

Hands and Knees

7. Starting Position: On your hands and knees with your knees about a foot apart and your hands on the floor in line with your shoulders.

- Shift your weight forward and backward while you are on your hands and knees. It's a very small movement—you may only move a couple of inches. In order to shift your weight forward, imagine that someone is pulling your head forward by a string. To move backward, imagine that someone is pulling your tailbone by a string.

8. Starting Position: Same as 7. (On your hands and knees with your knees about a foot apart and your hands on the floor in line with your shoulders.)

- Move your left leg to the side, keeping the knee bent, until it comes slightly off the floor, and then return to all fours. Try it on the right side with the right leg, and then alternate from one side to the other.

• After you're comfortable with the above exercise, include your head in the movement. Turn it to the right as you move your right leg and to the left as you move your left leg.

• If you are comfortable with your head and leg moving together, try moving them in opposition. As you move your right leg to the right, look to the left. As you move your left leg to the left, look to the right. This might feel strange so just take it slowly and easily and remember to breathe.

Standing

9. Starting Position: Stand with your feet about shoulder width apart and your knees slightly bent.

• Imagine that you are drawing a circle with your tailbone as you move your pelvis in a circular motion. Reverse directions. Remember, the circle can be very small.

• Widen your stance and allow your feet to turn out slightly. Draw circles with your pelvis in this position.

10. Starting Position: Same as 9. (Stand with your feet about shoulder width apart and your knees slightly bent.)

• Your belly will limit you on this exercise for sure. Reach to the ceiling with your arms and look up. Slowly lower your arms and head, and continue moving downward until your hands touch the floor and you're looking between your legs. (Your knees should be bent as much as necessary.) Press into the floor with your feet as you unroll to your starting position. Repeat but rest between repetitions to avoid dizziness.

11. Standing next to a chair, holding on to it with your left hand, gently swing your right leg forward and back. Your right knee should be bent and your leg should feel loose and easy, like a limp noodle. Keep the swing within your range of movement, not too high in the front or back. Turn around and swing the other leg.

12. Starting Position: Standing facing a wall, feet about 3 feet from the wall.

• Place both hands on the wall and step forward on your right foot. Bend your right leg and keep your left leg extended. Keep both heels on the floor. Hold for at least 15 seconds.

- Do the same exercise except bend your back leg also. Hold this stretch for at least 15 seconds.
- Repeat both stretches with the other leg.

Recommended Reading

Working Women

Brazelton, T. Berry. *Working and Caring.* Redding, MA: Addison-Wesley, 1987.

Ferguson, Trudi, and Dunphy, Joan S. *Answers to the Mommy Track: How Wives-Mothers in Business Reach the Top & Balance Their Lives.* Far Hills, NJ: New Horizon, 1990.

Paulson, Jane Hughes. *Working Pregnant.* New York: Fawcett Columbine, 1984.

Fathers

Greenberg, Daniel. *Confessions of a Pregnant Father.* New York: Avon, 1985.

Ostermann, Robert; Spurrell, Christopher; and Chubet, Carolyn T. *Father and Child.* Stamford, CT: Longmeadow Press, 1991.

———. *Fathering.* Stamford, CT: Longmeadow Press, 1988.

CHAPTER FOUR

Class 4—Week 38

What's in This Chapter

D-Day Overview

A Plethora of Procedures

Just Say Yes!

War Stories

Lamaze Breathing: Pushing Contractions

Work Issues: Carrying Both Loads—
Meeting the Demands of Your
Job While Pregnant

Taking Care of Yourself:
Taking the Edge Off

Exercises

D-Day Overview

Many feelings come together when you realize you are actually in labor. You feel excited, surprised, a bit scared. You have a strong sensation of anticipation but also uncertainty. You may be exhausted—common enough for the last month of pregnancy—and you may feel that you aren't prepared enough for what lies ahead.

We believe we've prepared you for the physical part of delivering a baby. But there are still many unknowns: What do you do when you arrive at the hospital? What's going to happen first? Can you have medication if you need it?

In this chapter, we'll give you an overview of what typically happens from the moment you enter the hospital or birthing center until your return home. If you're having a home birth, much of this will not apply. But again, you never know if a home birth will turn into a hospital birth, so skim through this section, too. Some of the information here will be somewhat familiar, but this overview is from a different perspective, one you'll be glad to have.

Checking In

A typical normal delivery begins in the admissions department of the hospital or birthing center during your first stage of labor. If you are preregistered, you stop at the admissions desk for a few minutes to make sure that all your paperwork is in order. You are given an identification bracelet, are asked to sign a consent form for the delivery (if you haven't already done so), and are then escorted upstairs to the maternity floor. Remember, if you haven't preregistered, you or your coach will be faced with about an hour of filling out forms, or you may be sent to the maternity floor by yourself, leaving your coach behind to do the paperwork. Again, we encourage you to preregister!

On the Maternity Floor

If you are being admitted to a hospital or birthing center, this floor is where you will be spending at least the next 12 to 48 hours, depending on the length of your labor and delivery and the facility you have chosen. If you didn't take a tour of your facility beforehand, you might want to check out the floor before you settle in—if you're in any condition to do so.

Most maternity floors are divided into birthing and/or labor rooms, delivery rooms, postpartum room, a small kitchen area where you can store your champagne for later on, showers, sitz baths, and bathrooms, waiting room for family members, nursing station, doctors' lounge, and nurseries. If you did take a tour prior to your admission, you already know the lay of the land and will automatically feel more comfortable with the surroundings.

The nursing staff is there to support you and your coach, so if you need anything, ask for it. Nurses work one of three shifts (7 A.M.–3 P.M.; 3 P.M.–11 P.M.; or 11 P.M.–7 A.M.), someone will be assigned to you at all times. If the shift isn't too busy, your assigned nurse will be in and out of your birthing room constantly. If your coach needs to be relieved at any time, all she or he needs to do is ring your call bell and a nurse will respond immediately. Labor and delivery nurses are there to support both you and your coach.

Traditionally, your coach is the only person allowed in the birthing room with you, but some hospitals are now allowing a "relief" person also to be present; others allow your children to watch, providing they have been to children's childbirth classes. Other hospitals, like the one in the story below, have extremely open policies.

A woman about to deliver her eighth child decided she wanted all her children at the birth. Her oldest was in high school, the youngest were toddlers. She eventually decided that the toddlers were too young, but five of her kids were at the hospital for the birth, including the oldest daughter with her boyfriend.

When the doctor was reached, he was having dinner with his ninety-year-old mother. Knowing that his patient would probably deliver very quickly, he had no time to take his mother home, so he brought her to the hospital with him. She, too, was invited to watch the birth. The final count in the audience was twelve, and included the father, the five kids, one boyfriend, the doctor, the doctor's mother, and three midwives.

You may not want this many people around, but if you are taking videos of the birth, you will most definitely require at least one additional person, because the coach will be too busy for videos or pictures. Make arrangements beforehand for the camera person.

Labor rooms in the nineties look like your bedroom at home. The bed is still a hospital bed, but it looks like a standard twin bed, not the huge metal beds of yesteryear. However, these simple-looking beds are equipped with everything. Some have the call button right on the panel of buttons that raise and lower your bed and contort it into unusual positions. Some beds have phones connected to these panels. We recommend putting the phone to the side until you have delivered, and don't give out the number. You will go crazy if people are phoning in to see how you are progressing. Most medical equipment, such as the emergency cart, oxygen, gloves, and examining equipment, are hidden behind cabinets, but are available immediately if needed. In labor rooms in birthing centers, medical equipment (IVs and fetal monitors) is usually not in the room, but rest at ease—it's very close by.

Labor rooms are generally very quiet, which is what you need. However, they aren't soundproof. Closing your door and your neighbor's door will usually provide enough of a sound barrier, but you may still hear birthing noises from an adjacent room, which can be disconcerting. Bring your own tape player and music to help diffuse all outside noises.

The delivery room looks a lot different from your birthing room. Generally, a delivery room is very sterile looking, with a delivery table in the middle, a clear plastic bassinet for the baby, huge lights over the delivery table, surgical equipment on movable tables covered with sterile drapes, and lots of shiny medical tools.

I'm Here, Now What Do I Do?

First things first. Make sure you know where the call button is located. You and your coach may find it necessary to use it on numerous occasions. An emergency is no time to find out that you don't know where it is. Most call buttons are located right next to you on the bed.

Next, change your clothes. Some hospitals and birthing centers will allow you to wear your own nightgown, and some will request that you put on a hospital gown. Actually, many women prefer the hospital gown because they don't want to stain their own gowns. In a hospital, your coach may be asked to put on surgical scrub pants and top. Again, this depends on your hospital's policy. Many hospitals won't require your coach to wear a surgical outfit unless you are having a C-section.

After you've changed, your nurse will need to get some information from you. She'll ask you the length and duration of your contractions. Your coach should have the answers. She may ask you when you had your last bowel movement, and if you have urinated recently. She will take your vital signs and listen to the fetal heartbeat. She will then proceed to do an internal exam to see how dilated and effaced you are. This exam feels just like one at the doctor's office, only a bit more uncomfortable because you are in labor. Remember to do your breathing!

Your doctor will stop by to see how you are progressing and to check your records. At this time, he or she may decide to start an IV with pitocin, a drug that stimulates labor, but if things are progressing fine, you will be left on your own. From time to time, your nurse will come in and check your cervix to see how much more you have dilated and effaced.

If your labor drags on, they may hook you up to the fetal monitor. If you're in a lot of pain, you can have medication. Your nurse will give you medication intramuscularly or intravenously, or the anesthesiologist will give you an epidural (a regional anesthesia that numbs you from the waist down). If you need or request medication, this can help just enough to get you fully dilated and ready to push.

When Push Comes to Shove

As you move into the pushing, or second, stage of labor, if all is normal, you probably will be allowed to stay in the same room. This is to your advantage, because changing rooms or beds at this point can be very uncomfortable! However, if complications arise, your doctor won't hesitate to move you into a delivery room where all the equipment is available if needed.

Although it may seem that you will be pushing forever, the average pushing time is only one hour. Some women push the baby out in three pushes, but others take up to two plus hours. Just before the baby's head is delivered you may have an episiotomy (a surgical incision that enlarges the birth canal). The decision may also be made to use forceps or vacuum extraction. Both are procedures that help deliver the baby. Again, medication will be given if needed. After you push the baby completely out, you and your coach will have a wonderful feeling of euphoria and elation.

There's Still More

Here we are again at the third stage. You still have to deliver the placenta. You'll be exhausted from the birth, but you'll have a renewed sense of energy because you have the baby in your arms.

Remember, when it's all over, you and your coach will have about 1 to 2 hours alone with the baby. The nurses will want to take care of you and the baby during this time, and they can help if you have any problems breastfeeding or have any questions. The baby will be taken to the nursery to be washed, weighed, and examined. If you have a boy and want him circumcised, your pediatrician will do the procedure the following day.

You will be asked if you would like to urinate. You will *not* want to, but try anyway, so your distended bladder doesn't make your uterus lose its tone and become boggy (soft). The nurse will wash your pubic area and put on a new sanitary napkin and belt.

It's Almost Over Now!

During the first hour of the fourth stage, the nurse will come in about every fifteen minutes and massage your uterus to make it contract, so that you don't bleed excessively. This can be an uncomfortable process, but it's necessary.

The baby will be brought back into the room, and you can nurse if the baby is interested. Nursing helps to contract the uterus, and may make you feel as if you are having labor contractions (very mild), which you are. This is a sign that your uterus is contracting in size.

Going Home

Nobody wants to stay in a hospital any longer than necessary. If you have a low-risk pregnancy, you may be able to have an early discharge. If so, you and the baby will be released from the hospital or birth center after you have both stabilized (6 to 12 hours). Make sure that you truly feel well enough to go home.

If you are not an early-discharge candidate, you and your baby will probably be discharged within 24 to 48 hours, barring any complications. Usually you will have a visit from your doctor the morning of discharge and he or she will sign the papers, and your pediatrician will do the same for the baby. Most discharges occur between 10 A.M. and 12 noon. Make sure that whoever is picking you up has brought the infant car seat. The hospital will not let you leave without one, even if you live in New York City and don't own a car!

Unfortunately, the mother must be discharged before the baby on some occasions—premature birth, jaundice, and respiratory problems, to name a few. There are also situations in which the *baby* is discharged before the mother. Both of these are distressing, and you should know your options.

If you are breastfeeding, it is especially silly to be discharged because you'll need to feed the baby every two hours. Know the policy of your hospital. Perhaps you can work something out. In any event, don't expect your insurance to cover any extra stay you do arrange. Hospitals are not hotels. If you have to use one as such, you'll find that it's the world's most expensive. And if your baby is really premature or ill and has to stay in the hospital many days or weeks, you'll have to accept that, staying with your baby during the day but sleeping at home.

There are rare situations where the baby is discharged before the mother. A friend of ours had complications from her C-section that forced her to stay in the hospital longer than her baby. Another friend *almost* had to stay in the hospital longer than her baby. She had a fever the last hour of her labor, and the hospital's policy was that she had to stay another 24 hours. Since nothing was wrong with her baby, the baby was to be released. She and her doctor worked it out so that she could go home with her baby, but it wasn't easy. It's a terrible situation to be in, but hospitals only have space for those who need it, and insurance companies do not cover well babies.

A Plethora of Procedures

Once you check into the hospital, the staff might start procedures that you didn't expect. You might not even know why they are doing them or, even more important, whether you *have a choice* in the matter. Before you arrive at the hospital, you should know your hospital's and doctor's policies regarding certain procedures such as shaving, IVs, fetal monitors, etc. At a birthing center, some of these procedures are also available but because of their philosophy of "less medical intervention" they aren't used as often as in hospitals. We'll describe all the common procedures. However, you must check with *your* hospital or birthing center and *your* doctor to find out their specific policies.

Prepping

Most hospitals no longer require enemas or the shaving of pubic hair. However, with C-sections, they will usually shave your pubic area with your legs closed.

IVs (Intravenous Fluids)

IVs are rarely started as routine procedure anymore. However, you will have an IV started under these circumstances:

- If your labor is to be induced, you are given a drug to start your contractions. The drug will be introduced through the IV.
- If your labor becomes long and possibly unproductive, an IV will be started for hydration and augmentation of labor.
- If you are nauseated and cannot drink, an IV will be started to prevent dehydration.
- If you need to have a cesarean section.

Electronic Fetal Monitor

An electronic fetal monitor is an ultrasound device that sends and receives sound waves to detect the fetal heart rate. One will be used if:

- You have a high-risk pregnancy.
- You are being induced.
- You are having a long labor.
- Your doctor needs an assessment of fetal well-being.
- Complications arise.
- Other medical intervention is necessary.

The monitor has two straps, which are attached to your abdomen. The top strap reads the uterine contractions, and the bottom strap is an ultrasound, which reads the fetal heart tone. There will be a strip of paper coming out of the monitor, which shows the length and duration of your contractions.

Some women find it annoying to have anything on their stomachs. The monitor also needs frequent adjustment when you move or the baby moves. Some women find that their coaches pay more attention to the monitor than to them.

Another disadvantage of a fetal monitor is that it restricts your freedom to move around. This may cause discomfort and may slow your labor. When fetal monitors first came into use, women were

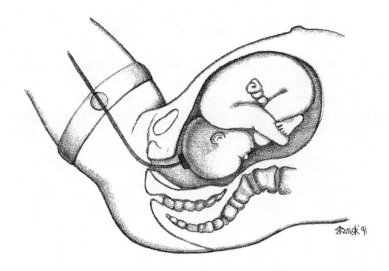

confined to their beds from that moment on. However, the monitors can be used intermittently, and this practice is in favor today. Typical is to "tune in" 10 to 20 minutes every hour. The rest of the time you may walk and move around. Know beforehand what the policy is.

Unfortunately, monitors are not always accurate. If the monitor gives a cautionary reading, other procedures will be done to verify the reading of the fetal monitor.

Internal Electrode

If you have meconium staining in your amniotic fluid, if more precise information is needed that is not being transmitted from the external monitor, or if further medical intervention is anticipated, an internal electrode will most likely be placed transvaginally onto the presenting part of the baby (the head) to obtain a reading of the fetal heartbeat.

The electrode, about the size of a small sewing needle, is placed barely under the baby's skin, and the procedure is similar to having a needle stuck under the skin of your finger. The electrode is attached to a long, thin wire, which is connected to a small box the size of a kitchen matchbox. The box is attached to your thigh with an elastic strap, which is similar to the fetal monitor band. They will leave the device in place and turned on during the entire labor.

The monitor lets your doctor know how your pelvic contractions are affecting the fetal heart rate, provides information should further medical intervention be needed, and is less restrictive than the external monitor.

It doesn't hurt you, either. You might feel as if you have a tampon string hanging between your legs. This may be annoying, but it will not hurt.

Episiotomy

An episiotomy is a surgical incision into the perineum (the region between the vulva and anus), either from the vagina toward the rectum (middle incision) or off to the side, a medio-lateral incision. Most women would prefer not to have an episiotomy—it doesn't fit their idea of a perfect birth—but 50 to 75 percent do have one. Talk to your doctor about his theory regarding episiotomies. And because an episiotomy enlarges the birth canal, it has other advantages:

- Speeding the delivery of the baby.
- Providing more space if your doctor is using forceps or vacuum extractor.
- Reducing the compression from the vaginal tissues on the head of a premature baby.
- Providing a straight incision, which is easier to repair than a serious tear.

Just Say Yes!

Prior to the 1980s, the Lamaze stance on medication was that women should not accept any medical intervention unless it was "a matter of life and death." The breathing patterns would take care of everything if they were used as taught in the Lamaze classes. In the 1980s, it was acknowledged that not only did medication help free many woman of pain, but because they were free of pain they were

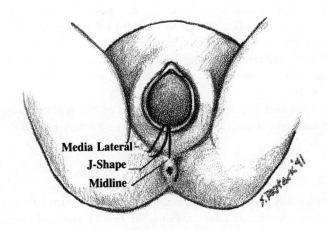

Episiotomy Incisions

more relaxed and therefore their labor and delivery moved much faster. Mothers cooperated a lot more, too. Lamaze instructors have adapted their teachings accordingly, and now explain the medications that are commonly used, and the pros and cons of those medications. It is still preferable for the mother not to use any medication if at all possible, because it is much healthier for both the mother and the baby.

Don't underestimate yourself during labor and delivery, but don't be a martyr, either! If you feel that you cannot handle another minute, let your doctor know. Just say yes. There's no point in suffering needlessly. If you are in too much pain, your ability to relax, which is related to your ability to dilate, can be hampered. If you are in too much pain, you may lose perspective on the situation. It's much healthier for you and the baby if you are as relaxed as possible and in control. Sometimes that means asking for medication. Don't feel badly if you need some. Think of it as a tool to help you get through labor.

Bertie had been in labor for over sixteen hours, and her doctor finally asked her if she wanted any medication to take the "edge" off. She valiantly said no. Her doctor grabbed her by her shoulders and told her not to be a martyr. She realized that the doctor was right, and agreed to an epidural immediately. Within minutes she was "in heaven" compared with the previous pain, and the rest of her delivery went fine.

The medications you might be given range from analgesics to anesthesias. Most would be administered through an IV, but they can be given orally, rectally, vaginally, or by injection, depending on the circumstances.

These drugs enter the bloodstream and affect the entire body— and your baby, by way of the placenta. Therefore, the timing of the administration of these drugs in relation to the time of birth influences the degree of risk and side effects to the baby.

The medications described below include the most common drugs used during labor and delivery. We've tried to give you enough information so that if and when it becomes necessary for you to request, or be given, any kind of medication, you and your coach will be as well informed as possible to make a decision.

Uterine Contraction Stimulators

Common Drugs Used: Pitocin and Syntocinon.

Purpose: Used to induce labor contractions, strengthen contractions, or control postpartum bleeding.

Normal Stage for Administering: First, second, and third stages and postpartum.

Common Situations for Administering: Your bag of waters has been broken for more than 12 to 36 hours and your labor has not started.

You are two weeks overdue.

Your contractions are not strong.

You have uncontrolled postpartum bleeding.

Disadvantages or Risks: Causes anxiety.

Causes edema (swelling).

Deprives fetus of oxygen with prolonged contractions.

Antidiuretic effect.

When improperly used can rupture uterus (very rare).

Efficacy of Drug: Dose takes effect within 15 to 20 minutes, and is adjusted gradually until adequate labor is established.

Sedatives

Common Drugs Used: Nembutal and Seconal.

Purpose: They do not relieve the pain but promote rest and relaxation and reduce anxiety.

Normal Stage for Administering: Prodromal labor (extended labor for days).

Disadvantages or Risks: Can prolong labor by interfering with uterine contractions.

Can cause disorientation and sleepiness.

Can build up in the fetal tissues and potentially cause respiratory depression and decreased sucking response.

Efficacy of Drug: Takes effect in 5 to 15 minutes and lasts approximately 12 hours.

Tranquilizers

Common Drugs Used: Vistaril and Phenergan.

Purpose: Reduces tension and anxiety. Vistaril and Phenergan are also used to reduce nausea and vomiting.

Normal Stage for Administering: During prodromal labor.

Common Situations for Administering: If you feel out of control.

If you are nauseated or vomiting.

If you are in pain that you cannot control.

Disadvantages or Risks: May cause drowsiness, dizziness, or disorientation

Changes in blood pressure and heart rate.

Blurred vision.

Dry mouth.

Efficacy of Drug: Works within 5 to 15 minutes and lasts 4 to 6 hours.

Analgesics

Common Drugs Used: Demerol, morphine (usually given with Phenergan or Vistaril), Nubain, Fentanyl, Stadol (these last three are the analgesics of choice at this time), Tylenol no. 3 or Vicodin (used for afterpains).

Purpose: Reduce the pain without a loss of consciousness. May promote relaxation between contractions and help promote the feeling of being in control.

Normal Stage for Administering: Usually given during the active phase of labor.

Common Situations for Administering: Used for pain during labor, discomfort after a cesarean, and to ease afterpains.

Disadvantages or Risks: Administration too early in labor slows down the uterine contractions.

Administration too late can make the baby sleepy and drowsy, and no drug can counteract this effect.

In mother may cause dizziness, euphoria, and nausea, and may lower blood pressure.

In rare cases, may depress the baby's respiration at birth.

Efficacy of Drug: Takes effect in 5 to 15 minutes and lasts 1 to 3 hours.

Regional Anesthesia

Locals, pudendals, epidurals, and spinals are four different types of regional anesthesia that you might be given. In general, they all produce numbness in the area injected or in the region of the body controlled by the affected nerves. They do not affect the mind or make you drowsy. They block pain impulses and are accompanied by numbness. They are given to relieve pain during active labor or birth.

Local

Common Drugs Used: Lidocaine or some derivative.

Purpose: Numbs the perineum and relieves pain during active labor.

Normal Stage for Administering: The second or third stage of labor.

Common Situations for Administering: Used primarily for an episiotomy or repair.

Disadvantages or Risks: None known.

Efficacy of Drug: Takes effect in 5 to 10 minutes and lasts for 1 1/2 hours.

Pudendal

Common Drugs Used: Lidocaine or some derivative (similar to Novocain).

Purpose: Numbs the vagina and perineum and relieves pain.

Normal Stage for Administering: Second stage of labor.

Common Situations for Administering: Forceps delivery.

Episiotomy or repair.

Disadvantages or Risks: Is only 99 percent effective.

May inhibit bearing-down reflex.

Efficacy of Drug: Takes effect in 5 to 10 minutes, and lasts for 1 1/2 hours.

Epidural Block

Common Drugs Used: Marcaine, Lidocaine, Fentanyl, or morphine.

Purpose: Numbs you from waist to knees. With an epidural, you no longer feel the contractions. (You *may* still be able to move your legs and push because it blocks the sensory nerves more than the motor nerves. You *may* still be able to feel pressure.)

Normal Stage for Administering: Active labor.

Common Situations for Administering: Often used for cesarean births.

Disadvantages or Risks: May slow labor. Pushing time may be 3 hours instead of 2.

Might feel like pins and needles.

May not be 100 percent effective.

Efficacy of Drug: Takes effect in 2 to 10 minutes and is usually given in continuous infusion.

Spinal Block

Common Drugs Used: Lidocaine.

Purpose: Numbs from breast level down.

Normal Stage for Administering: First stage and second stage.

Common Situations for Administering: Used for cesarean births.

Disadvantages or Risks: Possible drop in maternal blood pressure.

May have difficulty with urination after delivery.

May slow labor.

Possibility of a spinal headache. If you get a headache from a spinal, a procedure called a "blood patch" can be performed by the anesthesiologist, which alleviates the spinal headache almost immediately. The doctor will take some blood from the mother's arm and place the blood in the same spot that the spinal needle went in, and the opening heals itself.

Efficacy of Drug: Takes effect in 5 to 10 minutes, and lasts from 1 1/2 to 2 hours.

General Anesthesia

Common Drugs Used: Penthrane, nitrous oxide, and Forane or Isoforane.

Purpose: Produces a rapid loss of sensation and consciousness.

Normal Stage for Administering: Second stage.

Common Situations for Administering: Not a "common" procedure. Usually used in an emergency cesarean, if there are problems with the mother or the baby.

Disadvantages or Risks: May cause respiratory depression and changes in blood pressure and heart rate.

Increases the possibility of postpartum hemorrhage.

Efficacy of Drug: Takes effect in 1 to 5 minutes and lasts 4 hours or less.

War Stories

No two deliveries are alike. Our description of the typical hospital stay and the typical delivery are valuable guidelines, but you will not recognize the scenes in every instance. In order to demonstrate how similar yet how different things can be, we now will describe the very real deliveries of four women.

Denise's bag of waters broke on Saturday, but she felt no contractions. She called her doctor and was told to wait 24 hours. Nothing happened for two days, so on Monday her doctor asked her to come into the hospital to be induced. A pitocin drip was started and the contractions started coming hard and furious. Denise's contractions never slowed to a moderate pace, but remained hard and fast. They remained one minute apart for four consecutive hours. Her husband became so dizzy from doing the fast-paced breathing that he had to call in his mother as a relief coach until he could regain his composure. Denise held up better.

At 4 cm dilation, Denise was given an epidural, which made her feel wonderful, and she slept for a couple of hours, which was a relief, because she had been awake for over 48 hours at that point. At the time she felt guilty about the epidural but, in retrospect, realized that she couldn't have handled the pain any longer without it, and the sleep made it possible for her to push really well. Unfortunately, during transition Denise began vomiting. This made the contractions seem worse, but the vomiting subsided after an hour.

The Lamaze breathing was a lifesaver for her. Denise's initial reaction to the Lamaze class was that it was silly, but during labor she finally understood that it was worth the effort. A coach is a must, she concluded, because she panicked and lost track of her breathing on numerous occasions (although she did not get dizzy). Except during his dizzy spell, her husband was able to put her right back on track. She found she was most comfortable if she didn't open her eyes during the contraction, and if she listened carefully to her husband's voice while focusing on her breathing. She felt that the fetal monitor was a hindrance because she could see the contraction begin on the read-out, making her tense up before she could even feel it. Moving around helped minimize the discomfort; she didn't even consider getting into bed. However, when she had the epidural she had to be in bed. But by that time she didn't even care, as long as the pain was relieved.

Denise felt that the pushing was the most physical part of her labor, and luckily she only had to push for 20 minutes before her son was born. She had a small tear, which did not bother her for more than 24 hours.

Evan's labor started on Monday when she felt a trickle of fluid running down her leg. When she went to the bathroom she noticed blood on the toilet paper. She contacted her doctor, who told her that her membranes had probably ruptured—her bag of waters had broken—and the blood was from her mucus plug. Evan didn't notice any contractions, but she did feel "something" once every two hours. The following day Evan contacted her doctor. A sonogram showed that Evan did not have any amniotic fluid left. She was admitted to the hospital immediately. They started pitocin gradually at 8 A.M. and the baby was born at 10:30 P.M.

Evan's contractions were very regular and very painful, and the Lamaze breathing was quite helpful. Despite the complications, and despite the lack of a coach, she felt prepared for labor. Two shots of Nubain took the edge off. She was afraid, but the nursing staff was wonderful and made her feel as if she were with family. When the time came to push, Evan felt relieved to be doing something. One hour later her daughter was born.

Carol had preterm labor four weeks before her due date, and was placed on the medication terbutaline in order to control early labor. But she could not tolerate the anxiety and "hyper" feeling that resulted from the medication, so her doctor put her on complete bedrest instead.

When Carol was taken off bedrest, she immediately went into labor again. Her contractions were very regular at five-minute intervals, but not very strong. Carol had already been in the hospital twice with false labor, so her doctor was skeptical about the reality this time, but he advised her to check in to find out. Yes! This was the real thing.

Carol found that walking around helped her relax, but the shower was best of all—the only place she could truly relax. The nurses even took a fetal heart rate while she was in the shower. When her doctor arrived *he* didn't even ask her to step out while he listened with his stethoscope. Carol's husband was in the shower with her all the time. She suggests that all fathers be sure to take their swimsuits to the hospital.

When she was 4 cm dilated, Carol was given Nubain for the pain. The medication allowed her to relax, so her body was able to work with the contractions. Within two hours she was fully dilated. There wasn't a lot of resting time, so she was exhausted but still amazed at the power of the body when the time came to push. The pushing was a very powerful experience for her. She had the feeling that the body just pushed on its own, with or without her.

The mirror in the delivery room was huge—unlike the tiny one shown in the birthing film at the Lamaze class—so she and her husband could see the baby's head as it was emerging. However, Carol felt more comfortable with her eyes closed, so that she didn't really benefit from the mirror. Her husband did. The labor and delivery were ten hours—fantastic for a first time. She had a small tear, which was "really, really sore" for ten days. But she didn't care.

Sarah was two weeks overdue when her doctor decided to induce labor. At the hospital an ultrasound revealed that very little amniotic fluid remained. Sarah was placed on monitors and pitocin was started. Labor was moving along very well and the pitocin was stopped. The only voice Sarah could hear was her husband's. At 6 cm she was given an epidural, which made her feel terrific and helped her progress to the second stage. However, the baby was not dropping and his heart rate slowed to 50 beats per minute. Her doctor felt that the placenta was too old to handle the stress of labor. They prepared to do a cesarean, but Sarah had one last push and the baby dropped low enough for the doctor to grab him with the forceps. An episiotomy was performed prior to the forceps delivery.

. . . And so it goes with childbirth. There are over one million babies born every year in the United States, and each delivery is unique. Not a single one is 100 percent "textbook." Yours will not be, either. But why should it be? After all, we're not talking cloning here.

Lamaze Breathing: Pushing Contractions

You now understand and have practiced the slow-, moderate-, and pattern-paced Lamaze breathing techniques. It's time to combine the various breathing patterns with an imaginary pushing contraction. But first we'll warm up by reviewing the breathing techniques with a nonpushing contraction. As always, the quoted statements are for the coach.

1. **Contraction is starting. Take a deep cleansing breath, and move on to your slow-paced breathing (slow MOAN).**

2. **The contraction is getting stronger, so you want to use the moderate-paced breathing (inhale and ha 1–2–3).**

3. **Contraction is ending. Go back to the slow-paced breathing (slow MOAN).**

4. **Take a cleansing breath at the end of the contraction.**

Let's incorporate another breathing pattern into an imaginary contraction.

1. **Take a deep cleansing breath, and move right into your moderate-paced breathing (inhale and ha 1–2–3).**
2. **The contraction is really strong, so do your pattern-paced breathing (inhale—ha, inhale—ha, inhale—whroo).**
3. **The contraction is easing, so move back to your slow-paced breathing.**
4. **Take a deep cleansing breath.**

You are ready to begin pushing, so let's practice a pushing contraction. Remember, when you are practicing do *not* actually push. You could accidentally rupture your membranes.

1. **Contraction begins.**
2. **Breathe in and out, in and out, in and hold your breath to the count of 6.** (If you were actually pushing, you would try to push at this point).
3. **Press your chin onto your chest, place your arms on your knees, and imagine pushing the baby out.**
4. **As you feel the contraction end, take a deep cleansing breath. Stretch out your legs before another contraction begins. It's important to keep the blood circulating in your legs so you don't get leg cramps.**

Work Issues: Carrying Both Loads— Meeting the Demands of Your Job While Pregnant

Let's assume a best-case scenario: you have successfully announced your pregnant condition; bosses, fellow employees, everyone in the whole world couldn't be more delighted (they threw a big party); issues of maternity leave—well, there were no issues because your requirements and your employer's dovetailed exactly. In short, you live in the best of all possible worlds. Still, one question remains: can you do everything you used to do, or need to do?

In some situations, you and your peers on the job may have to make some concessions to your condition. But these don't have to be embarrassing or gratuitous or discriminatory. They can be common sense. And in many job circumstances, such as office work, you will not want or need special considerations at all. Here's what the American College of Obstetricians and Gynecologists has to say on the subject:

> The normal woman with an uncomplicated pregnancy and a normal fetus in a job that presents no greater potential hazards than those encountered in normal daily life in the community may continue to work without interruption until the onset of labor and may resume working several weeks after an uncomplicated delivery.

The guidelines go on to state that nonpregnant as well as pregnant women vary greatly in their ability to perform physically stressful work. Therefore, the guidelines conclude, it is not possible or even legally correct to make medical recommendations about the amount of lifting, for example, that is acceptable for pregnant women as a group.

However, the guidelines urge that special consideration be given to the physical hazards inherent in some jobs, including working at heights (on ladders, platforms, telephone poles, etc.) and operating certain heavy equipment and machines. An accident on these jobs would probably cause serious damage to the woman and the fetus, particularly after the uterus has enlarged out of the pelvis in the fourth month. Certain factory work, certain construction jobs, even some service-industry jobs, such as being a flight attendant, could require such possibly dangerous work. Many pregnant women may be uncomfortable in such jobs beyond midterm, but each pregnant woman must be individually evaluated as to her condition and suitability for a particular job.

In this section, we discuss physical and environmental hazards, major and minor, which you might encounter on your job. We suggest how to cope with those hazards as a pregnant woman. And obviously some of this advice also applies to general housekeeping work around the home that might require physical exertion or exposure to toxic chemicals.

Lifting, Pushing, Pulling

Your tolerance for lifting, pulling, or other physical exertion will depend on your particular fitness and strength, as well as the weight of the load handled and the circumstances. Sarah, a pediatric nurse, was engaged in various sorts of pulling and lifting every day on the job, but she worked until the very day she delivered. She knew and followed the rules for good body mechanics—stable support, use of the largest possible muscle groups, and so on—in all her lifting and pulling, but when she knew or even suspected that a particular job, such as moving especially heavy and immobile patients, was beyond her limits, she got help.

Teachers are always lifting boxes and pushing desks around. A friend of ours in her third month lifted a box in the classroom and immediately felt she had strained her back. She knew then she had reached a point where she needed help. Her supervisor understood completely and volunteered to send the custodian to help her finish that particular job and others with which she needed help over the following weeks. The neighboring eighth-grade teacher was happy to "loan" out a couple of her bigger students to help with heavy chores.

Getting Around

As the months pass, you may have more difficulty moving around. You will certainly have more difficulty moving nimbly. Your ever-increasing load up front affects stability and mobility. Your girth may start to get in the way. Such simple movements as changing from sitting to standing, climbing stairs, and bending become increasingly difficult as your pregnancy advances. You may have to find new ways of moving in order to accomplish the task at hand.

Kathy worked in a retail store and remembers getting stuck on the floor while she was restocking the lower shelves. She just couldn't get up. A security guard and a customer came to the rescue. But if those good Samaritans had not been handy, Kathy could have made it to her feet. Here's the technique:

- Lie down on your side, relax, and breathe deeply and calmly.
- Bend your legs and start pushing your upper body up with your arms.
- Gradually roll over onto your hands and knees.
- Place your feet flat on the floor one at a time.
- Press into the floor with your feet to come to a standing position.

You may have to climb several flights of stairs on the job or at home. Women have different strategies for handling this task, which only gets harder as the weeks roll by. One friend decided the only way she could make it up her four flights each day was to take them at a very slow but steady pace. She made sure that she was breathing deeply the entire time. Another woman found that if she did a little bounce when she placed her foot on a step this movement and visual image magically conveyed her onto the next step with much less apparent effort on her part. "Step-bounce . . . step-bounce": she recited this little mantra, silently or aloud, all the way to the top. Using your hands and semicrawling up the stairs is another possibility and worth trying.

Standing

If you have to stand in your work, take the opportunity to sit as often as possible, especially during the third trimester. You may realize very early in your pregnancy that you have to limit the amount of time you spend on your feet. Perhaps it is possible to do more of your job sitting than you had previously realized. For example, if you work at file cabinets for long periods of time, it's probably feasible to withdraw some of these files and work on them while seated at a desk or table.

When you do have to stand, raise one foot onto a footstool or box. This maneuver—beneficial for everyone, really—shifts your weight from your lower back onto your pelvis. The result is better support and less strain.

Flying

If flying is your job, you should know that the Supreme Court has ruled that for safety considerations you may be required to quit flying at a specific date in your pregnancy. For example, Delta Airlines requires their flight attendants to quit flying at twenty-four weeks and reassigns them to light duty.

If you fly as *part* of your job, your doctor may want you to curtail air travel six to eight weeks prior to the due date. But check with your doctor about how long you can safely continue to fly.

When you have to fly, make yourself as comfortable as possible:

- Reserve an aisle seat so you can get up and out as easily as possible. This is a good tip that's easily overlooked.
- Adjust your seat belt so that it rides over the bony pelvis and under your abdomen.
- Prevent dehydration by drinking plenty of juice or water.
- Wear good support stockings to help prevent swelling.
- Try to avoid sitting with legs crossed (as always).
- If you carry a small bag, place it under the seat in front of you and use it to elevate your feet.
- When you're out of your seat to go to the bathroom, walk up and down and get some exercise.
- Sit in the no-smoking section on intercontinental flights. (We naturally assume that you're not smoking while pregnant, and don't want to be around those who are. See below.)
- Carry a tennis ball in your bag and use it to massage your back. Slip the ball between your back and the seat and move your back from side to side. Start at the top, roll the ball back and forth, lean forward slightly to "drop" the ball slightly, roll back and forth, lean forward again, and so on. In a few minutes you will have given your back a surprisingly refreshing massage (a good traveler's tip for anyone). Your neighbor or the passenger seated behind you may wonder what's going on; that's their problem.

- Do other exercises to stimulate circulation and relax tense muscles. Several airlines explain such exercises in their in-flight travel magazines, but you can make up your own just as easily. All you have to do is "isolate" mentally any body part you wish, and then move it in as many directions and angles as possible. Give it a real workout. For example:

Head: Turn it left and right, move it up and down, and tilt it left and right. Combine all three and circle your head both left and right.

Shoulders: Lift them up toward your ears and let them drop. Move them forward and then backward. Circle them forward and backward.

Rib cage: Shift your rib cage to the right and to the left, then forward and back, then around in circles. Twist your upper body to the left and to the right. Tilt your torso to the left and to the right.

You can do similar movements with your arms, hands, pelvis, legs, and feet. If you're on a long flight, do *some* exercise several times an hour. The movements don't have to be large—they can't be, given the space confinements—but the more you move, the more comfortable your flight will be.

Smoking

Most women today have opted not to smoke during pregnancy, even if they were heavy smokers previously. (But if you are still smoking as you read this book, it's not too late to stop.) We know that chemicals in the smoke are absorbed through the lungs and then by way of the placenta, they may harm the fetus. This is common sense as well as common knowledge. Studies show that the chemicals in cigarette smoke affect the fetus in the following ways:

- Reduce the blood flow to the placenta.
- Increase carbon monoxide and decrease oxygen levels in the baby's blood.

- Increase the fetal heart rate.
- Increase the likelihood of low birth weight.

Unfortunately, some women who take great pains to avoid cigarette smoke work in a smoking environment. We don't want to sound preachy, but if you are one of these women, you might use the opportunity to discuss with management the benefits to all workers, not just pregnant women, of working in a smoke-free environment. The American Cancer Society and the American Lung Association are helping companies across the nation to change. If this is not possible in your workplace, ask if you can work as far as possible from any smoker. If that's not possible and your desk is very near a smoker's, explain the situation to him or her and see whether your fellow worker will cooperate by limiting smoking to areas away from you. Unless this person is really unfriendly, he or she will understand your concern, and might even take the first step after learning of your condition and volunteer to change.

You should also know that many cities and states have laws restricting smoking in public and private workplaces. States that restrict smoking in public workplaces are:

Alaska	North Dakota	Nebraska
Arizona	Ohio	Nevada
California	Oklahoma	New Hampshire
Colorado	Delaware	New Jersey
Connecticut	Florida	Oregon
Kansas	Hawaii	Rhode Island
Maine	Idaho	Utah
Maryland	Indiana	Vermont
Massachusetts	Iowa	Virginia
Michigan	Minnesota	Washington
New York	Montana	Wisconsin
New Mexico		

States that restrict smoking in private workplaces are:

Alaska	Minnesota	New York
Connecticut	Montana	Rhode Island
Florida	Nebraska	Utah
Iowa	New Hampshire	Vermont
Maine	New Jersey	Wisconsin

Each year the number of cities and states that are restricting smoking in the workplace grows. Check with your local government to see what the current smoking regulations are.

Hazardous Substances

The U.S. Occupational Safety and Health Administration (OSHA) has compiled a list of hazardous substances known to cross the placental barrier. A significant number of these substances can cause major birth defects and more subtle retardation and neurological changes with test animals. If a pregnant woman works with such substances on a regular basis, she should think seriously of switching assignments or taking an extended leave. You should avoid using potent pesticides, oven cleaners, paints, and solvents during pregnancy.

Substances known to affect the reproductive process are:

alcohol	diphenylhydantoin	methyl
aminopterin	ethylene dibromide	mercury
anesthetic gases	hexachlorobenzene	pesticides
busulfan	kepone	PCBs
carbon disulfide	lead	tobacco smoke
DDT	methotrexate	vinyl chloride
DES		

Substances known to affect the function of the placenta are:

carbon monoxide	mercury	pesticides
lead	organochlorine	cigarette smoke
cadmium		

It should be noted that until a recent Supreme Court ruling, many women did not have a choice in working with hazardous chemicals. At least fifteen major industrial corporations had fetal protection policies that banned women from certain jobs. The companies usually stated two reasons for these policies: they didn't want to endanger the health of the fetus, and they wanted to minimize their potential legal liability arising from birth defects. Historically, however, much of the expressed concern for a woman's existing or potential offspring has been a plausible-sounding excuse for denying women equal employment opportunities. According to one government estimate, these bans could make off limits to women as many as twenty million well-paid industrial jobs. These fetal-protection policies make a mockery of the Pregnancy Discrimination Act.

In 1991 the Supreme Court ruled in *U. A. W.* v. *Johnson Controls* that the company's fetal protection policy discriminated against women on the basis of their sex. According to the law, any fetal-risk decision is the responsibility of the prospective parent, not the employer.

Taking Care of Yourself: Taking the Edge Off

All of us occasionally get "stressed out" in normal, everyday living. When you're pregnant, especially when you're working, your stress level can skyrocket before you know it. To make sure that you stay as cool as possible, we recommend the following:

Be Realistic About What You Can Do

Common advice from pregnant women is *don't overdo*. We agree. The amount of work that pregnant women think they can accomplish is often way off the mark. Trying to do too much when you are pregnant only creates unnecessary tension and stress.

Make an honest assessment of what tasks, both at home and at work, are essential, and how you can accomplish them within the time available. What absolutely must be done, and what can wait? If you're really honest, more than half your "things to do" list could wait. This may be tough if you're a control freak, but it will be tougher if you continually try to do too much. Chill out, as your child will be saying one day soon.

Pregnancy can make working women feel they need to prove that they can pull their weight at the office. Well, you may or *may not* be able to do as much as normal. If you have to settle for 80 or 90 percent, the world (including your boss) will probably survive. If you usually leave the office at 7 P.M., leave at 6 instead. If you were a valuable employee or boss before your pregnancy, you will remain so during it.

Your husband can help with chores at home. Set up a routine of shared household responsibilities and *be specific* about who will do what and, if it's important to you, when it will get done. For the time being, some things may have to be less than spotless. When you bring the baby home, they *will be* less than spotless.

Watch Out for Too Many Changes

Be careful about making too many changes in your life at the same time you are having a baby. One monster change at a time is sound advice. This is common sense, but for some reason mothers and fathers often decide to make *other* big changes in their lives at the same time. Maybe the idea is to get it all out of the way. But try to wait until a few months after the baby has arrived before you make any radical changes.

Job and career changes are very common around the arrival of a new baby. Another mouth to feed often means more income is needed. Promotions or new jobs are sought. Parents evaluate their priorities and find that their present jobs don't fit into their new parental lifestyle. Maybe they want to change careers altogether.

Another person in the family means that eventually more living space is needed. Infants don't take up much space the first year or two, yet people put unnecessary and additional stress on themselves by moving to a larger residence in the midst of having a baby.

If you suspect you are caught up in too many changes at once, stop, freeze the frame, and ask whether you shouldn't slow down.

Get a Good Night's Sleep

Many pregnant women have insomnia. The cause is not known, but anxiety, fetal movements, muscle cramps, anticipation, the disruptions of sleep cycles, and cumbersome size must contribute to the problem. If you have insomnia, try drinking a cup of warm milk before bedtime, or try your deep-breathing exercises, which also encourage sleep. They may even put you to sleep. Relaxation breathing, soaking in a warm tub, a firm bed with pillows arranged to give you support, and regular exercise are all good remedies for insomnia. As we're sure you're aware, sleeping medications of any kind are not recommended during pregnancy.

Regular Exercise

We discussed the benefits and "how to"s of exercising in Chapter One. However, since it is one of the best stress relievers around, we couldn't leave it off this list.

Special Activities

Make time for activities that you enjoy and might not be able to do for some time after the baby is born. Take a long weekend with your husband. Go to the movies and out to dinner; visit friends.

Pamper Yourself

We'll go into a few details here, but they're probably not necessary. As busy and sometimes harried as many working pregnant women are, most figure out pretty early that they need some pampering to offset the hassles.

Pretend that you are at a spa. If you don't have time for the whole nine yards, give yourself any one of the following treatments:

Take Care of Your Swollen Legs and Feet: Start by elevating your feet to a level above your heart for 20 minutes. Then, while sitting, soak them for 15 minutes in a basin of warm water and softening bath oil or Epsom salts. Follow that with a quick, cool rinse, smooth on a cooling foot lotion with firm, massaging strokes on the balls of the feet, the instep, and the sides and bottom of the heel. Maybe you can even talk someone else into doing the massaging!

Take a Relaxing Bath in Warm Water: Always pleasant, but you *must* avoid the excessive heat of saunas, steam baths, mud baths, and hot herbal wraps. Raising the body temperature during pregnancy can cause birth defects in the fetus.

Soften the water with a soothing, fragrant bath oil, or simulate the carbonated springs of European spas with some mineral salts added to the bathwater. Follow up the bath with a body cream that seals in the moisture and helps keep your stressed and stretched skin supple.

Pamper Your Skin: A body rub can make dry skin feel soft again in just a few minutes. Body-rub creams, slightly grainy, slough off the surface layer of flaky, dead cells that can clog pores and leave the skin dull and rough. Simply smooth the cream onto the driest areas of your body and gently rub in with a circular motion. After you rinse and dry off, apply a generous coat of body lotion. However, it is important to use body-rub creams gently, and not more than once a week.

The traditional facial may be the ultimate way to pamper yourself. Some of the soothing effects of a salon facial can be reproduced in your own bathroom with a few simple ingredients. After you have cleaned your face, drape a towel over your head and lean over a basin of steaming water, 6 to 12 inches away. Ten to 20 minutes of this steam treatment will open your pores and help you relax. Follow the steam with a deep-cleansing mask, then rinse and apply either a moisturizer or a night cream.

You may be thinking, "Well, this all sounds great but it also sounds terribly expensive." But not every body cream costs $30. Believe it or not, many people feel Vaseline is the best moisturizer. You can whip up your own treatments at home, too. Several books have "recipes" for lotions, creams, and masks made from ingredients you have at home.

Exercises

Sitting

1. Starting Position: Sit with your legs together, extended in front of you. Make adjustments for your belly.
- Simply "walk" forward and backward on your sitz bones. Allow your legs to "walk" with you.

2. Starting Position: Same as 1. (Sit with your legs together, extended in front of you. Again, make adjustments for your belly.)
- Slide your right foot in toward your torso, keeping the whole foot on the floor, including your toes. Wrap your arms loosely around your right knee as your leg comes in. Allow your head and neck to bend toward your knee and your spine to round as your leg moves in. Release your arms and allow your leg to extend. Alternate legs. See how shifting your pelvis forward and backward can help you with this exercise.

3. Starting Position: Sit with your legs in a V, knees bent, feet flat on the floor.
- Let your hands rest lightly on your knees. Shift onto your right hip, allow your body to twist to the right until your left hip is off the floor. Allow your knees to move toward the floor as you shift and twist. Return to the starting position and then shift to the left. Be sure you include your head in this movement and look in the direction in which you are moving.

4. Starting Position: Sit with your legs folded in front of you or with the soles of your feet touching in front of you.
- Lift your shoulders toward your ears and then lower them.
- Move your shoulders forward and then backward.
- Make circles with your shoulders. Make them both forward and backward. Allow your arms to hang loosely. And, as you do this exercise, observe how your shoulder blades move too.

Side-lying

5. Starting Position: Lie on your right side with your knees bent.
- Gently roll to your left side. Feel free to use your hands to start

the roll. (If you are lying on your right side you would use your left hand.) When you arrive on the left side, take a few seconds to let every part of your body that is touching the floor really rest on the floor. Then roll back to the right side.

6. Starting Position: Same as 5. (Lie on your right side with your knees bent.)
- Make a 360-degree circle with your left arm, keeping your left hand on the floor all the way around. Allow your eye focus to follow your hands and move your upper body as necessary. Make circles in both directions and then roll to the other side and repeat.

Hands and Knees

7. Starting Position: On your hands and knees with your knees about a foot apart and your hands on the floor in line with your shoulders.
- Gently bring your right knee forward. As your knee moves forward, allow your head to move down toward your knee. Alternate legs.
- Slide your right foot backward on the floor until your right leg is extended behind you. Return to the starting position.
- Combine these two. Bring your right knee forward and take your head toward your knee. Then extend your leg to the back, keeping your foot on the floor and look toward the horizon. Alternate legs.

Standing

8. Starting Position: Stand with your feet about shoulder width apart.
- Let your arms hang loosely down by your side and gently twist your upper body from side to side. Allow your head to move with your upper body.

9. Starting Position: Same as 8 but take a wider stance.
- Rotate your upper body to the right, but as you do so, reach

with your left arm in the direction that you are rotating. When you rotate to the left, reach left with your right arm. Alternate from right to left.

10. Starting Position: Stand with your back against a wall and your feet 12 to 18 inches away from the wall.
- Slide your torso down the wall until your knees are bent at about a 45-degree angle. Stay in this position for 20 to 45 seconds.

11. Starting Position: Same as 8. (Stand with your feet about shoulder width apart.)
- Tilt your upper body to the left (including your head) as your raise your right arm toward the ceiling. Imagine you are hanging from your fingertips. Hang for 10 or 15 seconds if it is comfortable. Repeat to the opposite direction. Tilt right and raise your left arm.

Recommended Reading

Chubet, Carolyn T. *Pregnancy, Birth and Bonding.* Stamford, CT: Longmeadow Press, 1988.

Kitzinger, Sheila. *Pregnancy Day by Day.* New York: Knopf, 1990.

Trimmer, Eric. *Having a Baby.* New York: St. Martin's Press, 1988.

CHAPTER FIVE

Class 5 – Week 39

What's in This Chapter

Plan B

Feed Me!

Lamaze Breathing: Simulated Labor
and Delivery

Work Issues: The Challenge of Child Care

Taking Care of Yourself: Paying the Bills

Exercises

Plan B

Your delivery will not be picture-perfect, in all likelihood, because almost none are. In fact, many deliveries get quite involved. They turn out just as successfully as any other, but the road is sometimes a long and winding one. When labor begins, it's a very exciting time, and you shouldn't even be thinking about the "what if"s. You are focusing on your breathing and your relaxation skills. However, you should have a basic knowledge of the possible complications. Should something unexpected come up, you'll understand the medical responses without undo concern. The fears associated with these complications can grow out of all proportion if you aren't well informed. Just knowing what your doctor will do under different circumstances will ease the stress. Here's a closer look at some methods that might be used by your doctor should you require help, for whatever reason, in delivering your baby.

Forceps and Vacuum Extraction

Don't be alarmed if your doctor tells you he or she is going to use either forceps or vacuum extraction. Sometimes the baby simply cannot be pushed out, and your doctor will have to use one or the other. Neither option is ideal, but neither is threatening. Each is fairly common. The decision to use forceps or suction is usually made after the baby is at the +2 station, three-quarters of the way home but now needing a little help.

Forceps are a two-part stainless-steel instrument that are inserted into the vagina and applied to each side of the baby's head. Forceps came into common use in the 1920s to bring down the baby if the labor did not progress quickly enough. But since 1980 forceps have not been used as often.

However, they still might be used if:

- Your pushing is unsuccessful.
- You are exhausted.
- The fetus is responding poorly.

They may be beneficial because they:

- Rotate the baby's head.
- Protect a premature baby's head from prolonged pressure in the birth canal.
- Facilitate the birth of the head in a breech delivery, and allow for a rapid delivery if needed.

If your doctor decides on using forceps, you will most likely be given an epidural or pudendal block, numbing the vagina and perineum. Then you won't feel anything except the pressure of the forceps.

Many women have a forceps delivery without any other complications. They feel sore afterward in their perinenum, but this should be expected even if forceps are not used. In a typical forceps delivery, you will notice some bruising around the face or head area of your newborn. These bruise marks can be disturbing to the parents, of course, but they will go away within a week or so. We have previously related Sarah's story, in which the forceps and one last push were all that stood between her and a C-section. Sarah is a big fan of forceps.

A vacuum extractor is used to help the descent of the baby's head. Advantages of a vacuum extractor are that it can be used in a "malposition" case, or when the position is unknown. The extractor also requires less space in the vagina than forceps. Vacuum extractions have been in common use since the early 1980s, and have replaced forceps in many deliveries.

The extractor is a caplike device placed on the baby's head. A rubber tube extends from the cap to the vacuum pump, which creates a mild suction on the head. Your doctor will use the vacuum extractor to gently pull on the baby's head during contractions to help the newborn on its way. Afterward, the top of the baby's head may have a red mark, which will go away. Vacuum extractors may also cause bruising or swelling of soft scalp tissue. These will also go away quickly.

You should not feel anything unusual when the vacuum extractor is being used. You may feel the suction line lying against your thigh, but you will be busy pushing with each contraction and focusing on that.

The vacuum takes five to ten minutes to create the suction, and once that is accomplished, it isn't too long before the baby is delivered.

C-Sections: Emergency and Planned

Although every woman would like to have a vaginal delivery, it is not always possible. In 1988, nearly one million of the four million babies born in this country were delivered by cesarean section, commonly known as C-section. Thus the typical pregnant woman in America has a 25 percent chance of having her baby delivered through a surgical incision in her uterus. Breech babies account for about 10 percent of these—100,000 operations a year. Women over thirty-five are more likely to deliver by cesarean section (and this age group now accounts for nearly one-fourth of all births in this country).

It's important to have complete faith in your doctor, because you have to rely on that person to make the best decision for you and your baby if there is a problem that calls for a C-section. You may already know that you will have to have one. But even if you are not planning to have one, it's a good idea to know as much as you can about a C-section in case it is mandated at the last moment. Most doctors and nurses will encourage you to have a vaginal birth even if you believe you cannot go any further in the delivery, and indeed you should give vaginal delivery "everything you've got." However, if something happens that threatens your own or your baby's well-being, the doctor will not hesitate for a moment to do a C-section. It can save the day.

Here are the most common reasons for a cesarean delivery:

- Abnormal variations in the presenting part (which part of the baby is coming out first), such as:

  Face presentation

  Frank presentation (buttocks)

  Footling presentation (foot)

  Shoulder/transverse lie presentation (shoulder)

- Prolapsed cord: When the umbilical cord descends through the vagina before the baby, and causes the baby's oxygen supply to be greatly reduced.

- Abruptio placentae: When the placenta prematurely separates from the uterine wall, perhaps causing vaginal bleeding and/or abdominal pain, and also decreasing the baby's oxygen supply.

- Placenta previa: When the placenta is positioned across the cervical os (opening of the cervix), and as the cervix dilates the placenta separates from the uterus. Again, decreasing the baby's oxygen supply and causing excessive bleeding in the mother.

- Acute genital herpes: Can cause brain damage if the baby is born vaginally.

- Cephalopelvic disproportion (CPD): Means that this baby is simply too large to fit through the pelvis.

- Fetal distress: When changes in the baby's heart rate mean that its oxygen supply has been decreased.

- Prolonged labor: Contractions are of poor quality and dilation of the cervix and/or the descent of the baby is not progressing.

Prior to the 1980s, if you had a C-section for one delivery, all future deliveries would also be by C-section. However, times and techniques have changed. VBAC, vaginal birth after a cesarean birth, is very common. In fact, 50 to 80 percent of women who have had C-sections can have subsequent vaginal births.

Planned C-Section

If you and your doctor know beforehand you require a C-section, you can prepare for it and have some say in what happens. You have many options regarding surgery and delivery-room procedures, and you should discuss them with your doctor well in advance of the day of surgery. And on the day of surgery, make sure you refresh your doctor's memory of the decisions that have been jointly made.

Even if you aren't planning a C-section, please read these few paragraphs, because much of it applies to emergency C-sections as well.

Depending on your condition or the baby's condition, the following C-section decisions are negotiable with your doctor:

- Whether your delivery date will be determined by spontaneous labor, if possible.
- Whether the father can be present for delivery.
- Whether you may wear glasses or contact lenses during surgery. This may seem like a strange subject, but if you have bad vision and depend on your glasses, you might want to wear them so your first sight of your baby is not a blur!
- What medication will be used.

- What type of anesthesia (spinal, epidural, general)
- What type of medication is offered following delivery (analgesics)
- What types of incisions (horizontal or vertical) and closures (staples or suture)
- Whether any restraint of arms is used. Most women object to any kind of restraints, and fortunately they are no longer in common use. Be sure you discuss this one with your doctor.
- Whether the doctor will describe to you the surgery as it is happening.
- Whether a screen is lowered at time of birth or whether the baby is lifted above the screen.
- Whether the mother and the coach can touch the baby immediately after the cord is cut.
- Whether you and the father hold the baby after birth. This may sound silly, but sometimes everyone gets so carried away with the moment that they forget about the mother and father. This does not happen often, but it has happened. Don't be afraid to speak up if you have not been offered the baby to hold within a few minutes.
- Whether the baby is in recovery with the parents, if his or her condition permits.
- Whether the baby is breastfed in recovery, condition permitting.
- Whether routine admission of the baby to a neonatal intensive care nursery can be waived or shortened, if his or her condition permits.
- If the baby has a long stay in the neonatal intensive care nursery, may the parents visit, hold, and care for the baby (to promote bonding of parents and baby).
- Whether the mother may breastfeed in the nursery, or send in her own milk.
- Whether the mother can use beltless sanitary napkins (to avoid a sanitary belt, which irritates the incision).

C-Section: Step by Step

Let's go through a hypothetical cesarean step by step, starting with the prep work that is involved and ending with your recovery at home. The procedure is the same in most respects whether or not the C-section is planned, but we'll point out certain differences between emergency and planned. Of course, the main difference between planned and emergency (besides not being able to prepare for it) is the speed at which everything happens.

Prep Work: For most planned C-sections, you will go in the day of the surgery. In the past, the hospital staff wanted you in their care the night before, but now they simply instruct you not to have any food or water after midnight, and show up the following morning.

Once you are admitted, they will do some blood work, take your vital signs (blood pressure, temperature, pulse, fetal heartbeat), shave the top of your pubic area (including all the pubic hair visible with your legs together), start an IV, and insert a catheter into your bladder (which will stay there until you can urinate by yourself after surgery).

While your nurse is consulting your chart, she will make certain that your signed consent form is attached: if it isn't, another will be presented.

An anesthesiologist will come in and speak with you prior to surgery. Make sure that you are both in agreement regarding the type of anesthesia. Of course, in planned C-sections this choice should have been determined in advance.

With a planned C-section, all of this prep work takes about an hour. If you are having an emergency C-section, you will have an IV started, catheter inserted (or not, depending on the urgency), and will be given a general anesthetic—all in about ten minutes.

In the Delivery Room: When you enter the delivery room, you may be taken aback for a few moments by the surgical garb that your doctors and coach are wearing. This can make you feel distant from them and from the birth of your baby. But everyone in the delivery room is usually in an upbeat mood because they want to be there to see your new baby and to support you and your coach.

You will be washed with an antiseptic solution, which you will not feel, due to the spinal's numbing effect, and a sterile sheet will be placed over your abdomen. A low screen is put across your chest, which will prevent you from seeing the actual procedure.

This drape prevents you from seeing your stomach and from breathing on the incision, but it allows you to watch the doctor and see the baby as soon as it is born. Most doctors will lower the drape or hold the baby above the drape, so that you can see the baby (listed as a negotiable item, but almost all doctors will cooperate with your wish to see the newborn *immediately*).

Very few women want to be completely knocked out for the birth of their babies, even if they are having C-sections. If you have planned your C-section, you will have decided what type of anesthesia you want. Most women have an epidural or spinal. If yours is an emergency C-section, you might have either of these, or even a general anesthesia. Before beginning the operation, the doctor will make sure that the anesthesia has taken effect. You will not feel any contractions after you are anesthetized.

Your doctor can make two different types of incisions, and it is important for you to understand the differences, because they affect your options for future pregnancies. The first type of incision is called the transverse incision, or "bikini cut," the most common type. This incision is made horizontally just above your pubic bone. With the transverse uterine incision, it is possible to have a future vaginal delivery.

The second type of incision is the midline incision, which is made vertically from your fundus (the top of the uterus) to your pubic bone. This type of incision is done in emergency situations, and it usually isn't possible to have a future vaginal delivery.

Whether you have a bikini or a midline cut, your doctor will make two incisions. The first one will be through the abdominal wall (skin, fascia, fat, connective tissue). After this incision, the doctor will move your bladder out of the way and then make the second incision into the uterus.

The amniotic fluid is suctioned out of the uterus and the baby is gently lifted out. Immediately, the baby's mouth and nose are suctioned, just as with a vaginal birth. The actual birth comes a mere five to ten minutes after the beginning of the operation. After the delivery, the rest of the procedure takes about half an hour or more. The doctor will clamp the umbilical cord and give the baby to the pediatrician. The mother is given oxytocin to stimulate uterine contractions and make the placenta separate from the uterine wall. The

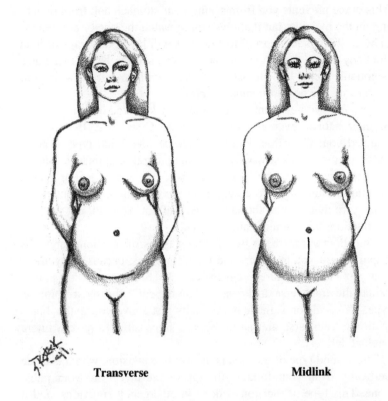

Transverse   **Midlink**

placenta is manually separated and removed by the doctor, and the uterus and abdomen are thoroughly inspected.

Then the uterus and abdominal fascia are sutured with absorbable suture material, and the skin is closed with nonabsorbable suture material, clamps, or staples, which will be removed before you leave the hospital.

Some women say that they feel pressure or pulling on their abdomen when their doctor is making the incisions, delivering the baby, removing the placenta, or closing the incision. If this happens to you, try to use your slow-paced breathing pattern to alleviate some of the discomfort.

After the Delivery: Once the baby is born, the nurse will take it over to a plastic or metal bassinet. The nurse and the pediatrician or

144

nurse anesthetist will check the baby over to make sure its color is good, and they will administer oxygen or clean out the nose and mouth if necessary. This is the same routine treatment as with vaginal delivery. After they have made sure that the baby is fine, they will bring it over to your husband or coach, and you can both share in the joy of this wonderful new being.

After the delivery, you will be washed and taken to the maternity recovery room, where your vital signs will be checked quite often, along with your uterus. If you have had general anesthesia, you will want to ask for some medication before they start massaging your uterus. If you have had a spinal or epidural, you will not feel anything for an hour or two. When you are "stable," they will move you into your room, where the baby will be with your husband or coach.

Your dressings (bandages) will be checked, and you will be given pitocin intravenously to make your uterus contract. Your IV is usually left in for at least 24 hours. Your dressings will be checked frequently and your IV will be removed once you begin passing gas or the nurses hear bowel sounds, signaling that your body is "waking up." Your catheter will be removed 12 to 24 hours after surgery.

You can expect four types of pain after C-section surgery: pain around the incision, uterine cramping, gas pain, and pain under the shoulder blades where air has been trapped under the diaphragm through your open incision. Do not hesitate to ask for medication to relieve any kind of pain.

Most women do not want to take deep breaths after surgery because it is uncomfortable. However, taking deep breaths really helps keep your lungs healthy, and promotes good circulation during this recovery phase.

After you are admitted to your room, begin moving your legs by bending one leg at a time. Keep one leg straight and bend the other leg at the knee. This will help you prepare for getting out of bed the first time.

Once you are allowed out of bed, the best thing that you can do is walk around and get your body in motion. The walking helps to alleviate a lot of discomfort that you may have with gas. These pains can be worse than the cramping, so get up and move as soon as possible. Try to stand straight and tall when you are walking. This will seem quite difficult the first couple of times, but it's better exercise, and will become easier.

Ask a nurse for assistance the first few times that you get out of bed. Occasionally, women become very dizzy and lightheaded, and even faint. When you first get up, you will also feel a gushing of fluid, which is the normal flow of blood after a delivery. Make sure you are wearing two pads to prevent major leaking.

Breastfeeding can be uncomfortable because of your incision, but it doesn't have to be. One of the most comfortable ways of nursing after a cesarean is to place a pillow over your stomach. You can rest your arms and baby on the pillow without hurting your incision. Another method is to hold the baby in a "football hold" while you are sitting up in bed. Place a pillow underneath the baby so you don't have to lean over to put your breast in his or her mouth. This position allows you to snuggle the baby close to you without much discomfort.

You will probably be back home with your baby within three to four days of delivery. Every hospital and insurance company is different, but that's the average stay for a cesarean delivery.

Try not to overdo it when you arrive home. Fatigue will take a toll on you sooner or later. A Snugli, or the Andrea carrier, is a great way to carry the baby around, because it equalizes the weight of the baby so you avoid bending, twisting, or pulling your incision.

Some women and their partners feel disappointed that they had to have cesarean deliveries. Many women feel "unwomanly." The most important point to remember is that you and your partner set out to have a healthy baby by whatever means. Having a cesarean is no comment on your womanliness or on your abilities to be a good mother. Just the opposite, in fact.

Three "Plan B" War Stories

Beth never went into labor. Her bag of waters broke without any contractions occurring, so her doctor tried to induce labor with a pitocin drip. But it didn't work—no contractions—so he sent her home with directions to come to the hospital each day for a stress test. Too many "dips" in this test indicated that the fetus was having a difficult time during a contraction, so a C-section was mandated. Morphine was the anesthetic of choice initially, then a spinal, but Beth recalls asking her husband nevertheless, "You *are* going to have a vasectomy, aren't you?"

The baby was born with breathing problems caused by the early rupture of the membranes, but Beth and her baby went home after five days, both feeling healthy and happy.

Lynn began her pregnancy weighing 125 pounds and ended up at 198 pounds! She had a terrible time with fluid retention, obviously, but she also had an unusual medical history. She was a child of a DES mother and had scarring on her cervix prior to becoming pregnant. A routine prenatal checkup (between her thirty-eighth and fortieth week) revealed protein and blood in Lynn's urine, and her blood pressure was literally off the chart. Her doctor put her in the hospital on the spot. He administered prostaglandin to her cervix, hoping to induce labor, but that was not to be. A pitocin drip was started and two hours later her bag of waters broke and "big" contractions began. Unfortunately, they stopped after a couple of hours. She was given some morphine so that she could sleep through the night.

The following morning the pitocin drip was restarted and Lynn's cervix began dilating slowly. Her contractions were hard and centered in her back. An epidural was started and she went from 4 to 6 cm. But instead of progressing from there, her cervix closed back up to 4 cm because it was inflamed from the baby's banging its head on it. At this point, Lynn asked her doctor for a cesarean, and the doctor agreed.

The anesthesiologist gave her a spinal, but Lynn still had to do her Lamaze breathing throughout the procedure. What truly pulled her through the surgery, however, was her husband's getting right in her face to coach her through. Their boy was a healthy 6 pounds 14 ounces.

Lisa woke up at 2:30 A.M. with cramps. Labor? She wasn't sure. But within half an hour her contractions were five minutes apart and becoming more uncomfortable. Her doctor told her to head for the hospital. Dilated to 2 cm when she arrived, she was up to 4 cm after an hour of walking, as directed by the nurse. Then she went into the shower. After four hours she was dilated to 8 cm, and the doctor broke her bag of waters. Her husband urged her to do her breathing; she told him to forget it! A couple of hours later she was still at 8 cm, and the baby's head was still at −3 station. Not much progress after ten hours of labor. Then Lisa's doctor told her that the baby's head was swollen and he would have to do a cesarean. When the anesthesiologist came in to explain what he was going to do, Lisa told him she didn't care what he was going to do. Just do it. He gave her a spinal, and she delivered a beautiful 8-pounds-11-ounces baby girl! All's well that ends well.

Cesarean Prevention

Many people feel that there are simply too many C-sections performed in this country. If your doctor is suggesting a C-section and you would like more information on cesarean *prevention,* the following books are recommended:

Rosen, Dr. Mortimer, and Thomas, Lillian. *The Cesarean Myth.* New York: Viking, 1989.

Flamm, Dr. Bruce. *Birth After Cesarean.* New York: Prentice Hall Press, 1990.

Or contact:

The Public Citizen Health Research Group
2000 P Street NW, Suite 700
Washington, DC 20036
(202) 293-9142
Request: *Unnecessary Cesarean Sections: How to Cure a National Epidemic* (cost: $15).

The Cesarean Prevention Movement
P.O. Box 152, Syracuse, NY 13210
(315) 424-1942
Send a self-addressed stamped envelope.

The International Childbirth Education Association
P.O. Box 20048, Minneapolis, MN 55420
(612) 854-8660

Feed Me!

Nutrition is important—very important—for babies, and mothers, especially working mothers, spend considerable time deciding whether to breast or bottle feed. The use of breast milk is recommended for the first four to six months of life for full-term, healthy babies, but some women are unable to provide mother's milk. A mother must bottle feed if she has had breast-reduction surgery, if she has hepatitis, if her breasts are infected, or if she receives drugs that could adversely affect the baby.

Some mothers choose to bottle feed because their schedules interfere with breastfeeding. Some working women are separated from their babies for days or even weeks at one time. And many working mothers who start out breastfeeding during their leaves of absence find it physically and mentally impossible to continue to breastfeed once they have returned to work.

The main point to understand is that if you bottle feed your baby, for whatever reason, there is no need to feel guilty about it. Many mothers today don't know that bottle feeding was the standard just one generation back. Many if not most of today's mothers who are so adamant about breastfeeding were themselves bottle fed!

Bottom line: Mother's milk is important, but loving your baby and merely holding your baby close are much more important for the child.

Breastfeeding

If you plan to breastfeed, do some homework. Obtain a good book on the subject (several are recommended at the end of this chapter). Attend a LaLeche League meeting if you have any questions before the baby is born. This group may be a little radical for your taste, but they have excellent resources concerning breastfeeding. Most important, prepare your nipples six to eight weeks before your due date in order to toughen them up. Using colostrum from your nipples or a wet washcloth, rub your nipples at least one to two times a day. This will make the first feeding a lot less shocking.

The baby will usually be breastfed before it goes to the nursery (usually one and a half hours old). The baby should have the nipple, including much or all of the dark part of the nipple, in its mouth and should be compressing the ducts (where the milk is) behind the nipple. Both breasts should be used at each feeding to ensure complete emptying. This will also stimulate milk production.

The normal time on each breast is from 5 to 8 minutes, with a burp in between. The theory now on breastfeeding is to let the baby nurse as long as she or he wants to, on each side. However, should you have a real guzzler on your hands, most nursery nurses will encourage an initial time constraint within the norms, to prevent your nipples from becoming sore and irritated. If they do become irritated, gently rub lanolin or colostrum on them after every nursing, but make sure that you wash them with a warm cloth prior to the next feeding. Another option is a nipple shield, a soft plastic device that fits over your nipple. This protects it from actual contact.

For the first couple of days, the baby will not actually be drinking milk, but rather colostrum, which contains antibodies and is important for the baby. Your milk will then come in two to three days after the birth, and this is when your breasts will become engorged. They will feel hard and hot. If they become uncomfortable, take a warm shower and try to "express" the milk with your hand or a breast pump.

Sometimes when your milk "lets down" (starts flowing) you will feel pins and needles in your nipples. Your natural response will be to pull the baby off the nipple. We'll warn you not to do this because your milk will spurt all over the place, but your reaction will be so quick and so automatic the first few times that our warning probably won't do any good. When you see the milk spurting, you'll remember the warning.

Of course, breastfeeding is easiest if you can be with your baby all the time. If you don't work outside of your home, there's no problem. If you work, an ideal situation is when you can take your baby to work with you. Some working women have sitters close enough to work to bring the baby to the mother for at least one feeding a day, or the mothers can go to them on their lunch hours. However, very few working women have these options, and expressing milk becomes the next best thing.

Expressing Milk

If you plan on breastfeeding, expressing milk will enable you to be away from your baby and still give him or her the benefits of your milk. Expressing milk is easy if you have a good breast pump, a good introduction to what's going on, and some patience in the beginning.

Nursery nurses more often than not will take the time to explain the ins and outs of expressing milk. They have a wealth of information, which they will enjoy sharing with you. Many hospitals provide electrical breast pumps, so the nurses can easily demonstrate how to use one. In the specialized 1990s, lactation consultants are *the specialists to contact.* These folks can be contacted for any questions or assistance once you are home. Plus, we're going to provide a thorough introduction to the subject right now.

Buying or Renting a Breast Pump

The idea of a pump usually conjures up images of the gas station and some machine as large as you are. But, in fact, a breast pump is quite small and manageable. It comes with a bottle, bottle cap, nipple, nipple cover, bell and nipple adaptor, and an electric or battery-operated pump. Renting breast pumps is common around the entire country and it costs much less to rent than to buy. A manual breast pump will cost about $50 to $80 or $600 for an electric pump if you want to purchase one. The cost of renting breast pumps varies. Many are rented on a sliding scale, according to your income. Ask the nursery nurses or lactation consultants which brand they recommend and from whom to purchase or rent in your area. But before you do either, investigate to see if the breast pump you have in mind meets the following requirements of a good and efficient device:

- Has automatic suck-release-relax cycles to simulate a baby's natural sucking action and prevent excessive prolonged suction on your breast.
- Can be used for double pumping to cut time in half and also raise prolactin (a hormone that stimulates lactation) levels.
- Offers adjustable vacuum to your comfort level.

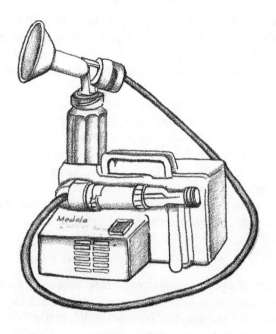

- Does not irritate or pull on your nipples (verified by friends or nurses).
- Has a nipple adaptor for the areola (the dark part of the nipple) when it is not getting enough pressure.
- Comes with a bottle so that the baby can be fed with the same container used to express. This helps prevent possible contamination caused by transferring the milk from one container to another.

How to Do It

Whether you are a learner or an experienced "pumper," try to find a quiet place and do a few relaxation exercises before you begin. Imagine your baby nursing or crying. This will allow you to "let down." A warm shower or warm compress on the breast also helps.

Make sure that you wash your hands thoroughly before expressing. The breast and nipple should be cleaned with water. Soap or other drying agents will dry and crack your nipples. And remember that all parts of the breast pump that come in contact with the milk should be thoroughly washed and sanitized (all parts washed in *hot* soapy water) before you begin.

Many women get frustrated initially with pumping, which only compounds the stress and negates the "let down" factor, which in turn compounds the stress even more. This vicious cycle can be avoided if you understand going in that a few weeks will be required to be really proficient at using any pump. If you get frustrated during this "breaking-in" period (or any other time, for that matter), simply put the pump down, walk away, relax, read a book, and then after you have calmed down, try again.

The other major problem you might have with expressing milk is nipple irritation. This can be caused by your pump, your technique, or nipple care. Make sure that after expressing you coat your entire nipple area with lanolin or Masse cream, which soothes the area and prevents drying, cracking, and irritation.

The basics of expressing milk can be described in five steps:

1. Do some gentle massage of the breast before you begin.

2. When first learning, nurse your baby on one breast while pumping on the other. The nursing will encourage milk flow. If the baby is unavailable, do your deep-breathing exercises and visualize nursing your baby.

3. Place the bell/cup (largest part of the pump) on the breast, centering on the nipple. If you have trouble getting a good fit with the bell, try using the nipple adaptor, which is made specifically for that problem.

4. Turn the suction valve clockwise until the suction pulls the nipple and areola into the bell. Use the suction-release button frequently to give a rhythmic sucking to the breast, as a baby would.

5. Continue to express until the flow of milk diminishes on one breast. Every mother is different, so the collection time can vary from 5 to 15 minutes per breast. You might feel that you are not getting enough milk at first, but as time goes on you will learn the best way to express for you. You should be able to collect 1 to 2 ounces with each pumping session.

Expressing Milk and Working Away from Home

Expressing milk takes extra effort for the working mother. You might as well acknowledge that in the beginning. If you want to start getting the baby used to the bottle before you are absent on a regular basis, you should use the breast pump to express and store for later use. If you can pump one to two ounces each day, that is more than enough. If that doesn't work out, you can supplement during the day with formula recommended by your pediatrician. You should have your husband or sitter give this bottle. Sometimes the baby will not accept a bottle from you, because he or she can smell the breast milk and knows your touch.

When you return to work, and if you are pressed for time in the morning, you can nurse the baby and use the breast pump on the other breast to have a fresh bottle for the sitter. And if your sitter can refrain from giving the baby a supplemental bottle an hour before you come home, you can nurse as soon as you get home, and you will have time to relax and the baby time to be close and cuddle. Often the baby will want to nurse frequently during the night.

While you are at work, you can express conveniently with a breast pump in the office lounge, a private office, or ladies' room. Find a quiet place away from the office activity, and try doing relaxation exercises before you begin. However, you may find that you agree with our friend Joy, who thought it was too much trouble to try to express milk at work. She coordinated her nursing so that she only had to express one bottle of milk per day and was able to do that at home.

Storing Expressed Milk

Breast milk must be stored very carefully. It is the perfect food for growth, both for babies *and bacteria.* The milk must be expressed into a sterile container. It can be stored in a refrigerator for use within 24 hours, or it may then be frozen for up to 2 weeks in a freezer. For longer storage (3 to 6 months), it must be frozen at 0 degrees Fahrenheit (colder than your refrigerator's freezer).

Store only 2 to 3 ounces of frozen milk in a single bottle, because once you have thawed the milk, you cannot refreeze it or even re-frigerate it. It must be used or discarded. Therefore, it's better to thaw two smaller bottles than to throw away a large quantity of milk the baby could not finish.

Do not add fresh warm milk to frozen milk. This would, in effect, defrost some of the frozen milk. Either freeze the new milk sepa-rately, or refrigerate it fully *before* adding it to the frozen milk, thus preventing defrosting.

To defrost the milk safely, hold the bottle under cold running wa-ter, then gradually warm the water until the milk is defrosted. It can then be warmed in a pot of water, but make sure it doesn't get too hot. Microwaves are not recommended because the milk heats very quickly and can be dangerously hot in 30 seconds. Parents can and should avail themselves of every convenience possible, but mi-crowaving milk is not one of them. It's too risky.

Bottle Feeding

If you have decided to bottle feed your baby, you will be faced with several decisions, including what brand of formula, what kind of bottle, and what kind of nipple to use. I know the last two don't sound very important, but when your baby won't take the bottle, it just may be he or she doesn't like the kind of nipple you have cho-sen. We certainly don't pretend to know what kind of nipple or bot-tle your baby will accept, or what kind of formula your baby will like or tolerate, but we can share information about the kinds avail-able and factors to keep in mind.

Formulas are either milk-based, as are Similac and Enfamil, or soy-based, as are Isomil and Prosobee. Some pediatricians don't want to wait for a reflux reaction (throwing up) to a milk-based for-mula, so they put newborns on soy-based formulas. Recent studies have shown that a soy-based formula, when compared to a milk for-mula, does *not* reduce the onset of allergies. Please discuss the choice with your pediatrician before you leave the hospital, and be ready to discuss it again if your baby has problems.

For babies who have asthma, eczema, or severe hay fever, or both of whose parents have documented food allergies, an "elemental" formula made from the protein hydrolysate is available. (If such an allergy-risk child is breastfeeding, the mother should avoid milk products, peanuts, and eggs in her own diet.)

Some mothers prefer using bottles with collapsible plastic bags because they think the bags reduce the amount of air that a newborn swallows. However, many physicians feel that the air that causes discomfort does not come from the bottle but from air in the nasal pharynx and oral pharynx that is gulped during normal swallowing.

Ultimately, your bottle-feeding choices may be your child's choices. One mother we know used formula for each of her three children. Each baby started off on Similac but was quickly switched to Isomil when an allergic reaction set in. This woman tried all the major nipple brands—Playtex, Gerber, Nuk, and Evenflo—and each baby selected a different one. (None liked the Playtex nurser, but lots of other babies do.) Her son was a "gobbler" and liked the Gerber nipples with three holes. Her first daughter liked to take her time and preferred the Evenflo with one hole. Her new daughter likes the Gerber during the day and the Evenflo at night. (To avoid popping off cap after cap in search of the appropriate nipple, this mother color coded the bottles.)

Lamaze Breathing:
Simulated Labor and Delivery

Now it's time to lay out an imaginary labor and delivery, and to practice your three breathing techniques within this context. In the early years of the Lamaze work, there was a clearly defined "division of labor" for the three different kinds of breathing. Each was to be used at a certain point in delivery. That philosophy has changed, and most Lamaze teachers now urge their pupils to experiment and feel free to use any of the breathing techniques at any time during labor. We also feel this is correct. Therefore, in your practice sessions between now and the actual delivery, make up a lot of different combinations. Coaches, this is primarily your responsibility. You'll be in charge of establishing the breathing. Start using your imagination now, during these practice sessions.

First Stage

Early Phase

Contraction example #1: **You didn't sleep beca~~use you were un~~comfortable and the baby was kicking all night.**

1. **Stand up. The contraction is easy.**

2. **Take a deep cleansing breath in through your nose and out through your mouth.**

Talk your partner through some slow-paced breathing.

3. **Do your slow-paced breathing. In through your nose, M-O-A-N out.**

4. **We'll do four more. In through your nose . . .**

5. **Take a deep cleansing breath in through your nose out through your mouth.**

6. **Contraction ends.**

Contraction example #2: **You have been sitting in the tub for one hour (bag of waters has not broken) and an easy contraction begins.**

1. **Take a deep cleansing breath.**

2. **Move on to your slow-paced breathing. In through your nose and M-O-A-N out. Repeat five times.**

3. **Take a deep cleansing breath.**

4. **Contraction ends.**

Contraction example #3: **You are at the hospital, at –1 station, 80 percent effaced, with 3-minute contractions, and dilated 3 cm. You are in bed, attached to a fetal monitor, and you don't like being in bed.**

First Stage

Early Phase

Contraction example #1: **You didn't sleep because you were uncomfortable and the baby was kicking all night.**

1. **Stand up. The contraction is easy.**

2. **Take a deep cleansing breath in through your nose and out through your mouth.**

Talk your partner through some slow-paced breathing.

3. **Do your slow-paced breathing. In through your nose, M-O-A-N out.**

4. **We'll do four more. In through your nose . . .**

5. **Take a deep cleansing breath in through your nose out through your mouth.**

6. **Contraction ends.**

Contraction example #2: **You have been sitting in the tub for one hour (bag of waters has not broken) and an easy contraction begins.**

1. **Take a deep cleansing breath.**

2. **Move on to your slow-paced breathing. In through your nose and M-O-A-N out. Repeat five times.**

3. **Take a deep cleansing breath.**

4. **Contraction ends.**

Contraction example #3: **You are at the hospital, at –1 station, 80 percent effaced, with 3-minute contractions, and dilated 3 cm. You are in bed, attached to a fetal monitor, and you don't like being in bed.**

1. **Contraction begins.**

2. **Take a deep cleansing breath.**

3. **Move on to the slow-paced breathing.**

4. **You are annoyed at being uncomfortable and want to get out of bed. FOCUS on your breathing.**

Take a tennis ball and rub her back gently as she moves through the contraction.

5. **The contraction is getting stronger. Do your moderate-paced breathing. Inhale and ha 1–2–3.**

6. **The contraction is subsiding, so go back to the slow-paced breathing.**

7. **Take a deep cleansing breath.**

8. **The contraction is over.**

Active Phase

Contraction example #1: **Your shoulders are tight, and you are 5 to 6 cm dilated. Try sitting tailor style with pillows propped up behind your back.**

1. **I'm going to rub your shoulders, back, and neck, if that's okay with you.**

Talk to her calmly as you massage her.

1. **Contraction begins.**

2. **Take a deep cleansing breath.**

3. **Move to the moderate-paced breathing, inhale—ha 1–2–3. Let's do three of these.**

4. **The contraction is getting harder, so move to the pattern-paced breathing, inhale-ha, inhale-ha, inhale-whoo. That's good. Let's do three more.**

Contraction example #4: **A new contraction begins, and your bag of waters just broke. All of a sudden the contractions are two minutes apart and very strong. Get on your hands and knees with this contraction.**

1. **Contraction begins. Take a deep cleansing breath.**

2. **Go immediately to your moderate-paced breathing, version 2: inhale hee, inhale-ha, inhale whoo.**

3. **The contraction is easing up, and you move to the slow-paced breathing.**

4. **End with a deep cleansing breath.**

5. **I'm going to sponge you off before the next contraction. Is that all right?**

Second Stage

Pushing Phase

Contraction example #1: **Try using a squatting or ballet position for this contraction.**

1. **A new contraction begins. Take a deep cleansing breath.**

2. **Move to the moderate breathing: inhale-ha, count 1–2–3.**

3. **The contraction is getting more intense, so move to the pattern-paced breathing: Inhale-ha, inhale-ha, inhale-whoo.**

4. **The contraction is letting up, so move to the slow-paced breathing and take a deep cleansing breath.**

5. **I know you're tired and you want this to end. You're doing great. Just keep focused on your breathing.**

Contraction example #2: **Stand with your knees slightly bent. I'll get behind you and hold you under your arms.**

1. **A new contraction begins. Take a deep cleansing breath.**

2. **The contraction hurts and you begin to shake. Keep breathing. Here's your paper bag. Breathe into it.**

3. **Move to the pattern-paced breathing: Inhale-ha, inhale-ha, inhale-whoo.**

4. **The contraction is easing up, so move to the slow-paced breathing.**

5. **Take a deep cleansing breath.**

Contraction example #3: **With the next contraction you're going to feel the urge to push but the doctor wants you to blow instead.**

1. **Contraction begins. Using your pattern-paced breathing, take three deep breaths. On the third breath blow as you exhale.**

2. **Contraction ends. Take a deep cleansing breath.**

Contraction example #4: **With the next contraction, you can pretend you are pushing. Bite a washcloth while you pretend you are pushing. It will help you focus.**

1. **Contraction begins.**

2. **Start your pattern-paced breathing. Take three deep breaths, hold the third one and count to six. (Remember, you're holding your breath instead of pushing.)**

3. **Contraction ends. Take a deep cleansing breath. Rest for one minute. Use one of your relaxation techniques or try to sleep.**

Work Issues: The Challenge of Child Care

Finding good child care is a prerequisite for returning to work, and a growing number of companies, large and small, are coming to the aid of their employees. Employers have finally realized that good, dependable child care means good, dependable employees. Many companies have child-care resource centers, which provide basic information about specific options and facilities in the community. These centers often serve as a referral service as well. Some companies subsidize employee costs.

Some companies have on-site care, with fees on a sliding scale based on salary. Some have backup care for those "emergency" situations when primary care breaks down: the private caregiver is ill, the regular child-care center is temporarily closed because the boiler is broken, etc. Other companies provide emergency care for the child who is too sick to attend regular child care but not sick enough to justify your staying home. Again, such enlightened child-care policies are just good business: your work is presumably worth more to the bottom line than the cost of providing subsidized or emergency child care.

A growing number of companies offer participation in a reimbursement plan for dependent care. The U.S. Tax Code allows employees to set aside up to $5,000 in pretax income for dependent care. Employees usually contribute money monthly and then submit their receipts at the end of the year for reimbursement. A few companies are also directly reimbursing their employees for child-care expenses when employees must travel.

Even though you may have your company's help in locating and paying for child care, you still have to make the final decision. You have to decide what kind of child care you want. You have to evaluate any child-care facility, including your own company's, or any caregiver whom you are considering. To help you find the right care for your child, we've provided a list of basic questions that apply to most child-care situations and that need to be answered in order to assure yourself you have found the best care possible.

The truth is that placing young children in the care of another person can be just as anxiety-rich as pregnancy, or even more so. We have urged you throughout this book to plan ahead with your pregnancy, to be prepared, and to do the work. The same goes for setting up child care.

Evaluating the Facility

- Is the child-care facility licensed? (All states have licensing procedures. Don't hesitate to ask to see a current license. If you have any doubts about what you're seeing, don't hesitate to verify matters with the state agency.)
- Is the location convenient to your home?
- Is the location convenient to your job?
- Are *all* costs, including extras such as after-hours and emergency care, clearly stated and available in writing, and is the information immediately and politely produced? If not, look elsewhere.
- Are meals provided?
- Can you visit the center during regular operating hours before registering your child?
- Are the caregivers present in sufficient numbers for the children registered? A ratio of three-to-one is excellent, four-to-one okay (and common). Anything less is suspect; keep looking.
- Do the caregivers teach in addition to caring for the usual basic needs?
- Do the caregivers have a policy about discipline?

Evaluating the Caregiver

What are the caregiver's qualifications? Are you invited to check the caregiver's references? You must check these references, and you should also account for any "holes" in them. Those lost six months in 1987 may have been a bad situation you would want to know about.

- Is the caregiver:
- Warm and friendly?
- Relaxed and patient with the children?
- Able to deal with each child as an individual?

Does the caregiver:

- Perceive play as important to children's growth?
- Listen to the children?

- Encourage the children to express themselves?
- Comfort crying children without implying that they shouldn't cry?
- Seem to be actively involved with the children, rather than sitting by passively?

Finally, and very important, does the caregiver seem to enjoy caring for the children?

Evaluating the Program

What do the children do all day? Are most of the following activities taking place when you visit? (Many of these are irrelevant for newborns, but your child may well be with the caregiver or in this child-care center for quite a few years. Besides, they speak to the general quality of the child care offered.)

- Creative play: look for crayons, paper, paints, clay, and other materials.
- Reading: look for books, some to be looked at alone, some to be read aloud by the caregiver.
- Play time: look for games and a wide variety of toys. For infants there should be toys that help develop sight, touch, and hearing.
- Music: look for musical instruments and records.
- Field trips: Ask if the older children visit nearby parks, libraries, museums, firehouses, and other places of interest. When they do, what goes on with the remaining younger children?
- Is there a place for outdoor play, perhaps a nearby park?
- Is television a large part—*too* large a part—of the planned activities?

Evaluating Health and Safety

Look carefully at this place where you are considering leaving your child. You will want to make note of the following:

- Is it clean? (Be sure to check the bathroom.)
- How are toileting and diapering handled?
- If meals and snacks are served, is the food nutritious? Does the food-preparation area meet appropriate standards for hygiene?
- Is there enough space for all the children? (In order to be licensed the facility has to meet certain standards of space, but also use your own judgment because the law might allow for tighter quarters than you would like.)
- Are there smoke detectors? Fire extinguishers? Alternate exits?
- Is there adequate heat, light, and ventilation?
- Is there a first-aid kit?
- Are all the medicines and poisonous substances locked up?
- Are there policies for ill children? Will the caregivers give medicine as prescribed to your child?
- Is there a physician consultant available?
- Is there a place for children to store their belongings?
- Does the equipment seem to be in good condition?
- Is there enough room for all the children to sit down at one time to eat?
- Are there provisions made for rest time? Cots?

Subjective Evaluations

Some of your assessments will be subjective. Think about the following:

- After you have been visiting for a while (or on a second visit), do your impressions stay the same?
- Do the children seem happy? Easily distracted? Overly eager and interested in seeing a visitor? Engrossed children who hardly give you a second glance are a *good* sign.
- Do the caregivers seem to be enjoying the work?
- Do you get the impression that parents are genuinely welcome when they deliver or pick up their children, or merely tolerated?
- Is there a nonsexist atmosphere (boys encouraged to play in the housekeeping corner, girls to play with trucks)?

Here's the bottom line in all these considerations, and the one question whose answer will dictate your decision: Do you feel intuitively good about leaving your child here?

Taking Care of Yourself:
Paying the Bills

You might think that filing for maternity benefits from your insurance company will be relatively straightforward and uncomplicated. Maybe. The only rule of thumb is this: check your policy carefully, consult with your agent if necessary, plan ahead. Just as many hospitals require preregistration, so many insurance carriers require prenotification, complete with estimated due date. A friend of ours in New York City discovered this almost too late; if she had waited until the last minute, she would have received less coverage.

Most insurance companies pay a fixed amount for physician and hospital services for a standard delivery with no complications, or a somewhat larger amount for a C-section. Likewise, almost all doctors and midwives charge a fixed amount. Your doctor's office will probably have you sign a form stating the amount that you will be billed for a normal delivery or for a cesarean delivery; your insurance company will take care of that portion of the fee, and your doctor's office will bill you for whatever is left over. Your hospital charges will not be quite so fixed in advance, because they'll charge you for every last bandage. But the hospital can give you the general range of charges; if your insurance covers, say, 80 percent, you'll know beforehand your out-of-pocket expense. There will be other, fairly minor, charges, including lab work, and these will probably be sent directly to you.

Health Maintenance Organizations (HMOs) seem to be easier to work with than private insurance. They normally charge a set fee for each visit to the doctor ($5 is common) and a nominal flat fee for the hospital ($25–$50 is common), and all the rest is covered.

Each system of insurance has its advantages, but in any event, by the time you read this book, it's too late to change your coverage. A new insurance policy will not pay benefits for any preexisting or ongoing condition, including pregnancy. Families and women who are without insurance coverage must fall back on their own resources and, if they qualify, Medicaid. Check with your local social services administrators if you are pregnant and without insurance.

Exercises

Sitting

1. Starting Position: Sit with your legs extended straight in front of you.

- Slide your feet along the floor, bringing both knees in toward your chest. (Your belly will limit you with this one, too.) Allow your head to move downward and your spine to round as your legs come closer to your torso. Allow your arms to wrap loosely around your knees. Extend your legs into the V position, again sliding your feet on the floor along the way. Slide your legs in toward your torso and then slide them back out to the starting position, legs extended in front. Notice how rocking forward and back with your pelvis and rounding your spine can make this exercise easier.

2. Starting Position: Sit with your legs extended in a wide V.

- Turn your pelvis, upper body, and both knees to the right. (Allow your knees to bend as you twist.) Your weight will be on your right hip and your left hip will be off the floor. Return to the starting position and repeat on the opposite side.

3. Starting Position: Same as 2. (Sit with your legs extended in a wide V.)

- Gently take your head toward the floor, allowing your spine to round as you go. Go only as far as is comfortable for you, and be sure you're breathing. A few good sighs or long exhalations in this position feel really good.

4. Starting Position: Sit with your legs folded in front of you or with the soles of your feet touching.

- Tilt to the right with your upper body. Reach overhead to the right with your left arm and allow your right hand to rest on the floor on your right side. As you reach, keep both sitz bones on the floor. Stay in this position for several breaths. Change to the opposite side.

- With each arm extended horizontally to the side, draw small circles with your arms. Make circles both forward and backward.
- With your arms extended horizontally in front of you, draw small circles.
- With your arms extended vertically overhead, make small circles in both directions.
- With your arms hanging down by your side, make small circles. (If your hands drag the ground, bend your elbows slightly.)

Side-lying

5. Starting Position: Lie on your right side, knees bent.
- Lift your left leg toward the ceiling and then return to the starting position.
- Lift your left leg toward the ceiling, but as you do it, press into the floor with your right leg. Lower it back down.
- Keep your feet touching and move your left knee away from your right knee.
- Keep your knees touching and move your left foot away from your right foot.
- Repeat all of these on the other side.

6. Starting Position: Lie on your right side with your knees bent.
- Gently swing your left leg forward and back, but as you swing your leg backward, allow your body to begin rolling to the left. Continue to roll until you are lying on your left side. Repeat, swinging your right leg forward and back, rolling to the right as you swing your leg backward. Be sure to support your lower back when doing this one.

Standing

7. Starting Position: Facing the back of a chair, both hands on the chair, stand with your legs about 18 inches apart and feet turned out slightly.
- Bend your knees and lower your torso toward the floor. (Again,

168

in dancers' terms this is a plié in second position.) To return to the starting position, press into the floor with your feet. (As you plié, make sure that your knees are in line with your feet. If they aren't, adjust your feet.)

8. Starting Position: Stand with your feet slightly wider than shoulder's width, knees slightly bent.
   • Make horizontal figure eights in front of your torso with your right arm. Allow the rest of your body to move as much as it needs to. Do the same thing with your left arm.
   • Make figure eights with both arms simultaneously but start your right arm circling to the right and your left arm circling to the left.
   • Make figure eights with both arms simultaneously. Start both arms moving to the right.

9. Starting Position: Facing the back of a chair, with both hands on the chair, stand with your feet about shoulders' width apart.
   • Bend your right knee and lift your right foot off the floor (it doesn't have to be high). Hold your foot off the floor for several breaths. If you want to test your balance, let go of the chair but be ready to take hold again when you need to. Change legs and balance on your right leg.

Recommended Reading

Cesarean Sections

Baldwin, Rahima. *Special Delivery.* Berkeley, CA: Celestial Arts, 1988.

Flamm, Dr. Bruce. *Birth After Cesarean.* New York: Prentice Hall Press, 1990.

Richards, Lynn Baptisti. *The Vaginal Birth After Cesarean Experience.* Westport, CT: Bergin & Garvey, Greenwood, 1987.

Rosen, Dr. Mortimer, and Lillian, Thomas. *The Cesarean Myth.* New York: Viking, 1984.

Breastfeeding

Eiger, Marvin S., and Olds, Sally Wendkos. *The Complete Book of Breastfeeding.* New York: Bantam, 1987.

Kitzinger, Sheila. *Breastfeeding Your Baby.* New York: Knopf, 1989.

Child Care

Auerbach, Stevanne, Ph.D. *Choosing Child Care: A Guide for Parents.* New York: E. P. Dutton, 1981.

Brazelton, T. Berry, M.D. *Infants and Mothers.* New York: Delta, Dell, 1974.

Dombro, Amy Laura, and Bryan, Patty. *Sharing the Caring: How to Find the Right Child Care and Make It Work for You and Your Child.* New York: Simon and Schuster, 1991.

Fredelle, Maynard. *The Child Care Crisis: The Real Costs of Day Care for You—and Your Child.* New York: Viking Penguin, 1985.

Growing Child. A monthly newsletter timed to your child's age. 22 North Second Street, P.O. Box 1200, Lafayette, IN 47902–1200.

Leach, Penelope. *Your Baby and Child.* New York: Knopf, 1989.

Siegel-Gorelick, Bryna, Ph.D. *The Working Parents' Guide to Child Care.* Boston: Little, Brown, 1983.

Spock, Dr. Benjamin, and Rothenberg, Michael. *Dr. Spock's Baby and Child Care.* New York: Pocket Books, 1985.

Sweet, O. Robin, and Siegel, Mary Ellen. *The Nanny Connection.* New York: Atheneum Publishing, 1987.

CHAPTER SIX

Class 6–Week 40

What's in This Chapter

Last but Not Least:
Postpartum Changes and Care

Maternal Instincts Aren't Always Enough

Work Issues: Back to the Nine-to-Five

Taking Care of Yourself:
I Want My Body Back

Exercises

Last but Not Least:
Postpartum Changes and Care

When most people hear the word "postpartum" they think of depression. There is a relationship, no doubt about it, but postpartum manifests itself in other ways, too. You go through dramatic physical and emotional changes during the first six to eight weeks after you give birth. Some of these changes are practically impossible to prepare for and would be considered abnormal or unhealthy under ordinary circumstances. But your body is not "ordinary" as it recovers from giving birth and begins to return to an unpregnant state, so this unusual period is actually quite normal.

Afterpains Are Normal

It's normal to experience *afterpains*. They are the contractions of the uterus that hasten its return to a nonpregnant state, and they are not only normal but beneficial. They occur immediately after delivery, especially while breastfeeding. (The sucking releases a hormone called oxytocin, which in turn causes uterine contractions.) Women who don't breastfeed also experience afterpains, but they are less frequent. Women who have had more than one child seem to have stronger and more frequent afterpains.

These usually disappear after the first week. But to lessen their effect until they disappear, try placing a warm blanket over your stomach and do your relaxation exercises. A full bladder will make the afterpains worse, so try to empty your bladder often.

Remember, normal afterpains are contractions of the uterus. If you have any other severe pain in your abdomen, legs, or chest, these could indicate postpartum complications. Call your doctor.

Uterine Changes

Your uterus should be contracted and firm after the birth, in order to prevent further blood loss, but it will require five to six weeks to return to its nonpregnant state. During this time, it is not uncommon for it to relax occasionally into a softer state, which you can easily feel. When it does so, press your hand into your lower abdomen and massage with a kneading motion. As you knead, you will feel your uterus become round and firm again. If it does not respond to the kneading, let your baby start breastfeeding. The sucking or licking action will cause the uterus to contract. If your baby isn't interested or if you aren't breastfeeding, either you or your partner should stimulate your nipples by lightly stroking them.

Check your uterus frequently, especially if you notice that it doesn't remain firm for more than a few minutes. If it remains soft and does not respond to massage of the breasts and abdomen, call your doctor.

Cervical and Vaginal Changes

Your cervix will shrink to its prepregnant size within six weeks. However, once you have given birth, the outer opening of the cervix does not regain its prepregnant appearance and remains somewhat wider. You won't be aware of the changes your cervix makes, and only your doctor will know that it looks different.

Your vagina, which was incredibly stretched out during delivery, will regain its tone. It may seem hard to believe that it will return to its former state, but it will. The labia will look larger and darker than before you were pregnant, and will retain their new size and coloration.

It is normal to have lochia—vaginal discharge. This is like having an extended period. The discharge starts out red and heavy for the first few days and then gradually decreases over three to four weeks. For the next week or two it will be brownish or pinkish in color. And then for another one to two weeks there will be a light yellow or white discharge. If it returns to a red and heavy discharge, if after the first 24 postdelivery hours you are soaking large pads in less than two hours, if there is passage of tissue or foul-smelling discharge, or if there is persistent passage of clots larger than a golf ball, call your doctor *immediately.* Any of these could be a sign of infection, overexertion, or hemorrhage, and require immediate attention.

Too Sore to Sit

It is also normal for your perineum and bottom to be sore for a few days, either from stitches or from the stretching during birth. You can put an ice pack on for the first 24 hours after birth to relieve swelling. Go (or send someone) to your pharmacy and purchase a foam "doughnut" to sit on. Carrying one around with you can be a real lifesaver!

Sitz baths (soaking in a warm tub) help, too. But don't bathe while you're in the tub or use any cleansing lotions that could cause irritation. Your "overextended" perineum is an excellent entry place for bacteria, and it's important to keep the water clean.

For that same reason, showers are definitely preferred for the first three weeks after birth. If you do not have a shower, purchase a hand-held shower attachment. They are inexpensive and fit on most bathtub nozzles. If a hand-held shower won't work for you either, take sponge baths.

To help keep your perineum infection-free, wash the area with warm water from a squirt bottle after each urination, and pat dry with a clean tissue, moving from front to back.

Breast Soreness

Initially, your nipples will be sore from your baby's sucking. It's a shocking experience at first, and it does hurt. When your milk comes in two or three days later, your breasts will be sore from that. It's normal for your breasts to continue to be a little sore until your baby has formed a nursing routine. But if you think your breasts are overly sore and you are extremely uncomfortable, call your LaLeche League or doctor for advice.

Some women experience engorgement of their breasts due to increased blood flow to the area and incomplete emptying during breastfeeding. This makes your breasts sore too. If engorgement or excessive swelling of the breasts does occur, expressing by hand in the shower may be helpful. Warm towels and frequent nursing should help, as well.

If you are not breastfeeding, your breasts will be sore because you have all this milk that is not being released. You will also have to put up with leakage. It will take at least a week for your milk production to stop. Most caregivers today do not give any type of medication to stop milk production, but some give medication immediately after delivery to suppress milk production. Ice packs and tight-fitting bras help prevent stimulation of milk production. Expressing your milk will *not* help, of course, but would only stimulate your breasts to produce more milk.

Elimination

Your urethra may swell immediately after delivery, making urination extremely uncomfortable or even impossible. However, during the first three days, it's important that you make yourself urinate at frequent intervals to prevent bladder infections. And, as mentioned above, urinating will help alleviate afterpains and help keep your uterus firm. If you have problems, try urinating in a sitz bath or in the shower. If this doesn't work, your doctor may order a catheter inserted into your bladder until you can urinate on your own (usually in 24 to 48 hours).

For the first weeks after delivery, it is normal to urinate in large quantities. You're drinking a lot of fluids (2 to 3 quarts a day) in order to replace fluids lost during labor and delivery, to help with your supply of breast milk, and to help prevent bladder infections. Simultaneously, your body is getting rid of the excess fluid associated with pregnancy. You can easily lose up to five pounds from water loss alone.

Usually, you will have your first bowel movement a day after delivery. Most women are quite apprehensive about this because they are sore and perhaps constipated. A cup of coffee or tea will stimulate your intestines. And Lamaze can still be beneficial: use slow-paced breathing during the bowel movement to ease any pain. Avoid constipation by drinking lots of fluids, eating lots of fruit, and walking. If you are still having problems with your bowels after a few days, ask your doctor to recommend a stool softener.

Vital Signs

Your temperature and pulse rate are good indicators of your well-being, and it's not normal to run a fever or have a high pulse rate. Your normal temperature is 96 to 99 degrees. If you develop a fever, drink lots of fluids and call your caregiver. If your temperature is over 102 degrees, take some Tylenol immediately and call your doctor.

Your pulse should not exceed 100 beats per minute. Take your pulse while sitting or lying down. If it is over 100, drink a lot of fluid and check it again in two hours. If it hasn't slowed down call your caregiver. If heavy bleeding is occurring at the same time, call your doctor immediately.

Diet

It's normal if your appetite isn't up to par, but it is important to focus on well-balanced meals. Try to continue with the same type of diet that you followed when you were pregnant.

If you are breastfeeding, you need more calories than normal. Spicy foods, cauliflower, and broccoli are not recommended for your diet until the baby is older, because they are all gassy foods for the baby. (Consult the specific diet recommendations of Chapter Two.) If you are breastfeeding—no alcohol. For generations, it was recommended that you drink a beer before nursing to help your milk production. Another old wives' tale! The truth is just the opposite.

Check with your doctor about continuing to take your prenatal vitamins. Many caregivers recommend a multivitamin plus an iron supplement.

Fatigue

It is normal to be tired. You're tired because you're recuperating from the incredible expenditure of energy required to give birth. You're tired because you probably didn't sleep the entire month before the baby was born and now you're not getting much sleep due to constant feedings. This is one childbirth rule to which there is never an exception!

To get as much sleep as possible, given the circumstances, follow your baby's sleeping schedule. The best routine for you and the baby is to feed the baby when it wakes, and put the baby back into its crib when you are done feeding. Nap when the baby naps, and get to bed early.

But if you're sleeping all the time, how will you ever get anything done? Let other people do some work, or let it wait. For example, if you normally cook all the meals, consider yourself on vacation. If your husband likes to cook, now's the time for him to take over the kitchen or pick up something on the way home. If your parents, in-laws, or friends are close by, you should ask for their assistance in providing meals or doing a few chores. However, if these relatives or friends are the sort who need to be entertained, you are better off without their "help."

During the first week you should only care for yourself and the baby. For the first couple of days it is wise to have someone other than the parents around. In this day and age, a lot of husbands are taking a week off from work to help around the house, which is absolutely wonderful for everyone. Some families hire nannies, nurses, or homemakers to help. These measures certainly allow you to recuperate a lot faster, but the hired help can be quite expensive ($250 to $500 per week). If you are planning on having a live-in nanny anyway, this is the time she should start her new position.

Whomever you bring in to help, just make sure she or he is someone you get along with. If your mother-in-law drives you crazy, this is not the week to try to straighten things out.

After the first week you'll feel like taking on more responsibilities. However, your activities and availability to visitors still need to be based on how rested you feel. And remember, your helpers are there mainly to give you time to rest, not time to race around like our friend Beth. When her mom arrived to help out, Beth decided to catch up on her office work and the many chores she had let slide the last month of her pregnancy. She began bleeding heavily, which her doctor attributed to overexertion.

Rest is essential for a total recovery. Nap during the day, think of ways to minimize your work, go to bed early, avoid lots of visitors, get help from friends and family, and exercise moderately.

Postpartum Depression

Over 60 percent of mothers experience some form of depression during the first week after the baby is born, usually around the sixth day. You may cry for no reason at all or at the silliest things, and/or you may withdraw from your husband and friends.

Most caregivers believe that postpartum depression is caused by a combination of the following factors:

- Tremendous hormone change.
- Breast pain and engorgement.
- Fears, anxieties, or guilt.
- A feeling of letdown, because you have built up these high expectations for at least nine months and now it's over.

- People are now focusing on the baby and not on you.
- You are disappointed about the type of delivery you had.
- You are disappointed with the sex of the baby.
- You are not prepared for the way your newborn looks—a red, wrinkled person with a pointed head. Not all that pretty, really. Shocking, even.
- You feel overwhelmed with the entire situation.

This emotion usually passes within a couple of weeks, but what can you do until then?

- Caring for the baby may alleviate some of these feelings.
- Communicating with your husband or friends is very important for emotional and physical support. Talk to other women who have been through it. Let your husband, friends, doctor know how you are feeling, and discuss it in great detail. Communicating relieves a tremendous amount of stress, and helps you have a better perspective on life. Sometimes just listening to yourself alleviates your worries.
- Relaxation and rest are extremely important in putting your fears and concerns in perspective. When you're tired you lose perspective, compounding your depression.

If your depression lasts for more than a few weeks or becomes unbearable, it is important to seek professional help. Contact the maternity floor at the hospital or your doctor and he or she will be able to refer you to a professional. Extended postpartum depression, although quite rare, can be a very serious situation and can lead to extended psychiatric care. You should be aware of the possibilities. If you are feeling out of control, please contact your physician immediately! Not seeking help will just compound the situation. You *can* be helped in this situation. There's no doubt about that.

Postpartum Sex

Many women are apprehensive about having intercourse after giving birth because they are sore, they are tired, or they think it will interfere with caring for their baby. You may have one or all of these feelings. They are legitimate apprehensions.

Most doctors recommend abstaining from intercourse for the first six weeks postpartum, but this is just a general guideline. When your stitches heal, your vaginal discharge stops, and you want to make love, go ahead. Remember that you can become pregnant even if you are nursing, so ask your doctor for his or her recommendation for contraception during this time.

Initially, if you or your partner feels any anxiety, try caressing, touching, kissing, and fondling without entry. Use K-Y jelly or contraceptive jelly for the first few times because your vaginal secretions will not be the same for a while, because of hormonal changes. You might assume a position on top so that you can control your partner's depth of entry. Doing Kegel exercises frequently, including during sex, will help you regain the muscle tone in the vagina and pelvic floor.

Women who are breastfeeding may find that sexual relations just aren't the same because their breasts are extra-sensitive, they feel that they should only be "used" for the baby, and they leak milk profusely during intercourse. Talk through these concerns. Wearing a nursing bra might help.

Follow-up Care

It is customary to have a checkup four to eight weeks after delivery to ensure that you are completely recovered. You will have a pelvic exam at this time along with a general exam. You may have a pap test, but this varies from doctor to doctor. Use this time to discuss any problems or questions that you have regarding yourself or your baby. Nursing, birth control, and sex are common topics of discussion during this checkup. But don't hesitate to ask your doctor any question or voice any concern you might have.

Maternal Instincts Aren't Always Enough

A friend called her on the second day home and she repeated, "She's here 24 hours a day, and she doesn't leave!" For this new mother, the responsibility of caring for another person *every hour* of the day and night was beginning to sink in. She was terrified. The first weeks of caring for a new baby can have such moments, but most of your time you'll be too busy feeding, changing, holding, and comforting your newborn.

New mothers will receive advice from many different people, and it is best to accept it graciously, but take it with a grain of salt. Much of the advice is either out of date or completely erroneous. Consider the following examples:

"Let the baby cry." Or "If you put the baby down for a nap, don't pick the baby up as soon as it cries."

Babies cry for a number of reasons: they are hungry, their diaper has to be changed, they are sick, something is bothering them, or they need love. They don't cry because they are trying to bug you. Use your common sense. If the baby cries for more than a few minutes (five maximum), pick him or her up.

"You feed that baby too much. You should only feed the baby every four hours."

The every-four-hours theory is now passé. Most pediatricians agree that you should feed your baby on demand, which means when the baby is hungry. You will have a calm, content baby if it is fed when its stomach is saying, "I'm hungry."

"Don't take the baby out of the house for the first month."

This is the ultimate old wives' tale! Most caregivers will recommend that you take the baby out for a walk after the first week, or when you are feeling up to it (usually by the second or third week).

So, if you have any questions regarding the care of your baby, ask your pediatrician. You want the best for your child, and your pediatrician will have the most up-to-date and accurate information and advice for you. And use your common sense. As your parenting expertise increases, you will learn to trust your instincts and your knowledge of your child. You will be less likely to let someone who does not know your particular baby and (probably) has no professional training tell you what to do.

A Baseline for Care

Much of your care is simply a matter of observing how your baby looks, feels, and responds. But if you've never had a baby before you need a baseline standard. For example, if you've never seen a newborn baby, how do you know if yours looks normal? How do you know if your baby is responding normally? Eating normally?

More than likely your baby looks, feels, and responds like most other babies, but just to make sure you know what to expect, and know when to be concerned, here are some general guidelines for newborns and their care.

General Newborn Appearance

Size

- 5–8 pounds
- 18–22 inches long

Head

- Possibly oblong from the molding during birth.
- Possibly swollen in the soft tissues of the scalp after delivery (caput succedaneum) owing to the pressure of the cervix on the head. This is common in long labors and will disappear within 48 hours.
- Possibly swollen scalp caused by bleeding under the skin—cephalohematoma. This is usually absorbed within six weeks.
- Two soft spots on its head, one at the top and one at the back. Tough membranes cover and protect the tissues underneath, so you don't have to worry about touching them.
- If the baby had an internal fetal monitor, there will be a red mark on the scalp with some swelling. It will disappear within a couple of days.

Skin

- Color will vary according to racial background and state of activity. Newborns, regardless of race, are usually quite pink after birth and may turn red during crying or vigorous activity.
- For the first few days after birth, the baby's skin may turn yellow owing to excess bilirubin. This yellowness will fade away; exposure to sunlight through a window may be helpful. If the yellowness appears on the first or second day or increases rapidly, or the whites of the eyes appear yellow, call your pediatrician.
- You may also notice some red marks on the baby's face. These are called stork marks and will disappear within a couple of weeks.
- Mottling of the skin, rashes, peeling, and flaking are all normal unless accompanied by other symptoms. You can use lotion or baby oil. If pus is present with a rash, call your doctor/midwife.
- Fine, downy body hair called lanugo may be quite visible.
- The lotionlike substance vernix caseosa may cover the baby to varying degrees. The vernix protected the baby's skin in utero, and it is all right to let it soak into the skin gradually.

Hands and Feet

- Hands and feet may appear blue or feel cool to the touch, due to normal circulatory imbalance. However, the face and lips should never be blue. If they are, call your pediatrician immediately.

Eyes

- Crossed or wandering eyes are normal.
- The eyes may appear swollen or red due to the antibacterial solution dropped into the baby's eyes immediately after birth. This will disappear within the first week. If there is a significant amount of yellow or green discharge, call your pediatrician.
- Darker-skinned babies show their true eye color within a few

weeks, but fair-skinned babies may not develop their true color for weeks or months.

Breasts and Genitals

- Breasts and genitals might be swollen. There may be a slight secretion of fluid from the baby's breasts, which should not be touched, except when bathing. Girls may have a vaginal discharge, perhaps even tinged with blood, for three to five days. The mother's hormones transmitted through the placenta cause these reactions, which are temporary.

Umbilical Cord

- The umbilical cord will be dark brown and dry.
- It will drop off when the baby is one to three weeks old. (This can and usually does happen when you are changing the baby's diaper or cleaning the cord.)
- Cleanse the cord and the area around it with cotton balls or cotton swabs and alcohol, whichever your doctor recommends. Do this several times a day (easiest around diaper change).
- When you are diapering the baby, make sure that the top of the diaper does not cover the cord area, which will keep the *cord dry*. Fold the diaper under so it does not touch the cord. If you notice any foul smell or discharge, call your pediatrician immediately.

Other Newborn Information

Elimination

- Black and tarlike bowel movements called meconium stools occur within the first 24 hours. The next several stools, loose and greenish brown, are transitional. By one week of age the breastfed baby will be having yellow, soft or liquid stools, anywhere from one with each feeding to one a week. The stools of formula-fed babies tend to be darker in color, more formed, and stronger smelling.

183

- Once the colostrum changes to true milk, the baby should have 6 to 8 wet diapers a day. Anything less should be noted and discussed with your pediatrician.

Eating

- Your baby should be fed on demand, 8 to 18 times per day, or approximately every 2 hours.
- Quantity, whether milk or formula, depends on the baby and the baby's size. They get what they need. If you are bottle feeding, start off with 4 to 6 ounces per feeding.
- After several months, average feedings drop from 10 or more to about 5 each day.
- If your baby is having problems sucking, call your pediatrician or your local LaLeche League.
- A newborn's sense of taste and smell are highly developed, and within a couple of days can differentiate between sweet and sour.

Sleeping

- After an initial period of alertness for a few hours after birth, most babies become sleepy and quiet for extended periods, and remain so for the first one or two days. This is a normal reaction to the stress of labor and birth, and adjustment to extrauterine life. After the first few days, the baby will have more wakeful moments. To the dismay of their mothers, some babies require little sleep during the day, but sleep all night. You cannot "schedule" their sleep patterns. They will let you know when they are tired. However, try putting the baby down immediately after feeding, and see what happens. Obviously, if the baby cries for 5 minutes, it wants to come out and play. Try again in a little while. Fresh air is a great sleep inducer. Every baby is different, and so are their sleep patterns.

Movement

- You may notice that the baby's arms and legs fling out violently when she or he hears a loud noise. This is called the startle reflex, and will go away around three months of age.

Hearing

- Sounds that are lower soothe the baby, sounds that are high-pitched startle the baby. A baby will turn its head to follow a sound.

Sight

- The newborn can see objects well up close, but not at far distances. It can see best at 7 1/2 inches away. Babies prefer curved lines and patterns.

Vital Signs

- Checking your baby's vital signs is not a normal at-home procedure. The signs are taken constantly in the hospital nursery for the first 24 hours. So unless you have had a home birth, or an early discharge, disregard the following information. However, if you have given birth at home, you will need to check your baby's vital signs every couple of hours for the first 24 hours. So please pay close attention.

Temperature

- The baby's normal rectal or axillary temperature should be between 97 and 99 degrees. To take a rectal temperature, place the baby on a changing table on its belly; with one hand spread the buttocks and insert the thermometer. The thermometer should have Vaseline or K-Y jelly on the tip, which will help ease the thermometer into the rectum. Insert the bulb until you reach the first numbers on the thermometer (approximately 1/4 inch). Leave in for 5 minutes and read.
- Cold can stress the newborn. In a medical facility, the room temperature is carefully controlled and monitored—not so in a home. If you have delivered your baby at home, or if you have taken early discharge, it is wise to take your baby's temperature frequently and adjust her or his clothing and the room temperature accordingly. The room temperature should be 80 degrees if

the baby is naked; reduce by 10 degrees for each layer of clothing you add. A knitted hat is one of the most effective ways of retaining body heat.

Respiration

- The normal range of breaths per minute for a newborn is 30 to 40. Count the rise and fall of the chest for 30 seconds and then double that number. A newborn's breathing is usually shallow, erratic, and snuffly. If the baby's nose or throat has enough mucus to be noisy, you may suction gently with a bulb syringe. Make sure you know what you are doing before you attempt this. It's easy to blow the mucus *into* the lungs and really cause trouble. Have your doctor/nurse/midwife show you first.

Pulse

- The normal range in newborns is 120 to 160 beats per minute. You can put your fingers gently on the baby's chest over its heart and count.

When to Call Your Pediatrician

Now that you have a baseline for your observations and care, we'd also like to give you some guidelines regarding when to call your pediatrician. If you observe any of the following signs, please call your pediatrician.

Temperature

- Rectal temperature is over 99 or under 96.
- The baby's temperature keeps changing, even when room temperature and clothing remain the same.

Respiration

- Fewer than 30, or more than 60, breaths per minute while resting.

- Labored breathing and grunting, retraction of the ribs, or flaring of nostrils.

Pulse

- Pulse outside the normal range of 120 to 160 per minute.

Elimination

- No passage of urine or stools in first 24 hours after birth.

Other problems

- Excessive sleepiness—sleep periods lasting longer than 6 hours after the first day.
- Hyperirritability or extreme reaction to ordinary stimulation like diaper changing, careful handling, etc.
- Jaundice on the first day.
- Poor feeding, none at all, or total exhaustion afterward.

Providing for Your Child's Safety

Most parents would agree that the safety of their child is a primary concern throughout their lives. Common sense goes a long way when making your child safe, but if you've never raised a child, you might need some outside help at first. We've provided basic safety information, which will give you a good safety orientation. However, many YMCAs, Red Cross chapters, and hospitals offer safety and first-aid workshops that you might also be interested in taking. Many books on the subject are on the market and are good to have on hand as references.

Bath Safety

- Check the temperature of the bathwater with your elbow. If it's too hot for your elbow, it's too hot for your baby.
- An adult should be present constantly while your baby is in the

bath. Wrap your child up and take him or her with you if you must answer the telephone or the doorbell.

- Keep one hand on the baby at all times during his bath.

Auto Safety

- Purchase a car seat that has been tested for a crash situation. Travel beds and lightweight household infant seats have no value in the car.
- Follow manufacturers' instructions for installing the seat and securing your baby or child in it.
- Always put the baby in a car seat when driving; never carry him or her in your lap.

Dangerous Objects

- Keep pins and other sharp objects, such as scissors and knives, out of the baby's reach.
- Plastic bags, plastic wrap, etc. should be kept away from the baby.
- Pick up buttons, beads, and hairpins from the floor. A baby can find the smallest bead on the cleanest floor.

Falls

- Remember that for the smallest infant, a bed with bars and/or a playpen is the safest place for the baby to be alone. Infants can wiggle and topple off a high surface, so never leave the baby on a changing table or in a crib with the sides down.
- Do not leave the baby unattended in an infant seat that is on top of anything.
- When you are busy, put the child in a crib or playpen as close to you as possible.

Burns

- Keep hot liquids, hot foods, and electric cords of irons, toasters, and coffeepots out of the baby's reach.

- When shopping for baby sleepwear, check to see that the garment has been treated for fire resistance.
- Check the temperature of formula and solid food before feeding the baby. Food should be lukewarm, not hot.

Toys

- Buy toys too large to swallow and without sharp edges or removable parts.

Crib

- Crib rails should be close enough together so that the baby's head won't fit through.
- Do not put a pillow in the baby's crib until he or she can roll over easily by himself or herself.

Miscellaneous

- Always place your baby on his or her side or abdomen after feeding, never on her back, so he or she won't vomit and aspirate stomach contents into the lungs.
- Wash all new clothes, bedding, etc., before putting on your baby.
- Pin diaper pins so that they open away from the midline of the baby. This way, if they open, they won't stick your baby.
- Never give the baby drugs not recommended by your physician.
- Keep detergents and other household cleaners out of cabinets that are low, or use locks.
- Prepare a list of emergency phone numbers including:

Emergency—911
Poison Control Center
Pediatrician
Fire
Police
Medical
Mother's office

Father's office
Neighbor

Work Issues: Back to the Nine-to-Five

Whether by choice or by necessity, you as a working woman have a job that amounts to a second life away from home. You have been away from that job for at least several weeks, perhaps several months. You might never have been away for a longer period, nor have returned after time off with as many mixed emotions. A lot has happened, to say the least, in your life, and now it's back to business as usual. The experience can be overwhelming—it probably is for women who have just had their first child—but it can also go rather smoothly. We highly recommend preparing yourself as much as possible.

Although it may sound silly, one of the most practical preparations is to check out the clothes in your closet. If you're returning to work shortly after giving birth, most of your nonmaternity clothes will not fit. You're probably sick of your maternity clothes and wouldn't be caught dead in them anyway. We're not suggesting you go out and buy a whole new wardrobe, but it is wise to think through the dilemma prior to 7:30 A.M. on Monday morning. Days or weeks ahead, find the time and the emotional energy required to try on everything in your closet in an attempt to find something that fits. You probably do have some clothes that either fit or can be made to. However you resolve the situation, do so before your first day back. You won't need a last-minute hassle over what to wear.

We also suggest you take a few "trial runs" away from your newborn. Your first day back at the office should *not* be your first day away from the baby. This may as well be stated bluntly: your initial feelings about separation from your baby will be your biggest hurdle in returning to work. Even if you desperately want to return to your career and work, it will not be easy because returning requires *leaving*. Trial runs away from your baby can help prevent your being emotionally overwhelmed on the first day at work. You'll have enough to deal with on the job. In addition, these practice runs will enable you to test your child-care arrangement and make certain that your travel times have been figured properly. Monday morning is not the time to learn that rush-hour traffic adds twenty minutes to the trip to the child-care center. Knowing that the logistics are well in hand will ease some of the anxiety about returning to work.

Call your boss and/or colleagues and remind them that you're coming back. You might even set up a lunch date prior to your return in order to get a head start on reestablishing your closest relationships. You can learn a lot in one hour! In addition, a lunch date with a good friend can steady you emotionally.

Be prepared for changes, for feeling out of it, and for being confused some of the time. If you've been away for a long time, a number of things about your job and company may have changed dramatically. It might seem like an entirely new job. But whatever happens, don't panic: give yourself time to adapt and to get things reorganized. Remember that you were doing well before you left, so you'll do well upon your return. And remember that you just successfully came through pregnancy and childbirth. Not many jobs pose greater challenges than that.

Taking Care of Yourself: I Want My Body Back

Many women who have just delivered turn attention immediately to getting back into shape. But that phrase is rather misleading, because if you ate nutritiously while you were pregnant and if you exercised regularly, you *are* in good shape—good physical condition, that is. But, like most women, you will probably still look four to five months pregnant after your baby is born, and your abdominal muscles will sag like elephant skin. So what most postpartum women really mean when they talk with conviction about "getting back into shape" is losing those extra pounds and toning up their abdominal muscles. And this can be done, but not overnight. Give yourself time. Most women require at least six months, perhaps an entire year, to get back their normal figures.

Let's talk first about those extra pounds. Many women are disappointed at how little weight they actually lose immediately after the birth of their child. Twelve pounds is the average loss, including the weight of the baby, the amniotic fluid, and the placenta.

The remaining weight, ten to twenty pounds, is all the fluid retained by your body, along with some extra fat around your hips, thighs, and buttocks that served as a reserve supply of energy while pregnant, and as help with milk production if you're breastfeeding. If you are nursing, an extra five or ten pounds will be with you until you wean your baby. When you stop nursing, or if you are not nursing and are ready to shed those extra pounds, they will disappear slowly if you follow a sensible meal plan. You can't expect to lose these remaining pounds overnight. In fact, you shouldn't try. Research indicates that crash diets are detrimental to losing weight in the long run. What you can do is:

- Choose low-fat foods.
- Choose moderate-sized servings.
- Eat plenty of fruits, vegetables, and other high-fiber foods.
- Drink 8 to 10 glasses of water a day (not including coffee, tea, and sodas).
- Avoid foods high in sodium.
- And remember that not all calories are the same: a calorie from a carrot is not the same as a calorie from a doughnut.

Exercise is the other requirement for losing weight and getting back into shape. Your abdominal and pelvic-floor muscles are the two areas that need immediate attention. If you have exercised regularly during your pregnancy, you are probably eager to resume your program. But check with your caregiver before you start doing any exercises, whether they're the ones we've provided in this book or your normal three-mile run.

Depending on your condition, you can return to exercise sooner than you might believe. Most women are allowed to start their Kegel exercises within hours of birth, thus addressing one of the two major areas that need special attention. The Kegel exercises help tears and episiotomies heal, they help reduce swelling of the perineum, and help restore muscle tone. You can probably take your baby out for a walk in the stroller as early as one week and resume your regular program within six weeks. But, again, check with your caregiver for a schedule.

Exercises

As we discussed earlier, your abdominal muscles will need lots of work postpartum. Most people think of sit-ups or "crunches" when they want to work on their "abs," but we're offering you more than sit-ups in this chapter.

Add two or three of these exercises a day to the ones you were doing prior to your baby's birth. But be sure you have your caregiver's okay to start any postpartum exercise program and be sure you're checked for abdominal separation. When you are given the okay, we still recommend starting with two or three repetitions and building very gradually. We also remind you to use your breathing to help you do these exercises.

Lying on Your Back

1. Starting Position: Lie on your back, knees bent, feet flat on the floor, hands clasped behind your head.

- Slowly lift your head off the floor, then gently lower it. Lift it only as far as it will easily move. There should be no discomfort.

2. Starting Position: Same as 1 but arms are down at the sides of your body.

- Lift your right leg and bring your right knee toward your chest. Return your foot to the floor. Alternate legs.

3. Starting Position: Same as 2.

- Extend your leg, keeping your foot on the floor as long as possible. Then slide the foot back to the starting position. Alternate legs.

4. Starting Position: Lie on your back, knees folded in toward your chest, feet off the ground.

• Alternately touch each foot to the floor and return it to the starting position.

5. Starting Position: Same as 4 but clasp your hands behind your head.

• Do the same exercise as 4, lifting your head with your hands.

6. Starting Position: Same as 4 but arms extended horizontally on the floor at shoulder level, palms down. Lie on your back, knees folded in toward your chest, and feet off the ground. Extend your arms on the floor at shoulder level, palms down.

• Drop your knees to the right until the side of the right leg touches the floor. Return to the starting position and drop your knees to the left. Alternate from right to left.

7. Starting Position: Same as 6.

• Swing your knees first right and then to the left. Go back and forth, imagining drawing a figure eight as you go.

8. Starting Position: Lie on your back, knees bent, feet flat on the floor, arms down at your sides.

• Raise your head off the floor and look between your knees. Press your elbows into the floor as you lift your head.

9. Starting Position: Same as 8.

• Do exercise 8 but continue coming up. Press your elbows, then your hands into the floor as you come up.

Recommended Reading

Bosque, Elena, R.N., M.S., and Sheila, Watson, R.N. *Safe and Sound*. New York: St. Martin's Press, 1988.

Chubet, Carolyn T. *Your Baby's Health and Safety*. Stamford, CT: Longmeadow Press, 1990.

Merenstein, Noel. *Baby + Life*. New York: Doubleday, 1990.

CHAPTER SEVEN

Common Questions

We have answered many of your questions in this book. However, we know you may have many more, because most pregnant women have an endless supply. And well they should: it's all new territory. So we have devoted this chapter to common questions that pregnant women ask. Some of the questions repeat material covered in previous chapters, but they are asked so frequently that we think they're worth repeating.

If you still have questions after reading this book, ask your doctor. Just because we haven't answered your question doesn't mean it's a stupid one and not worth answering.

What makes my legs and fingers swell?

You normally retain fluid during pregnancy, but too much fluid retention can be a sign of preeclampsia. Preeclampsia is characterized by a sudden and excessive retention of fluid, and rapid weight gain. Swelling can also be caused by the compression of the inferior vena cava, caused by the baby's pressure. Lie on your left side, and elevate your legs. If you have these symptoms, report them to your doctor immediately!

Will the stretch marks disappear?

Over time, they will turn from a red coloration to a whitish or silverish color, but they will most likely never disappear. Rubbing vitamin-E oil on your abdomen, hips, and breasts will keep the skin moist and supple, and, hopefully, prevent stretch marks.

What is the long dark line from my belly button down to my pubic area, and will it go away?

This line is called the linea negra, which is quite common and no cause for alarm. The line will disappear postpartum.

Will my breasts get any larger after the baby is born?

Yes, your breast size will increase approximately one full size. If you are planning on purchasing nursing bras prior to the baby's birth, it is wise to buy one or two bras one size larger. If you feel that the bra is too tight once you have had the baby, you can always increase bra sizes without having spent a fortune on bras that don't fit.

I am taking medication to prevent an early labor. Will it have any effect on the baby?

If you are concerned about any medication, or if you are having any side effects, please contact your doctor. Everyone is different, and many times health care may be individualized.

What can I do for my constant backache?

Pelvic tilts on your hands and knees are a real lifesaver when it comes to relieving back stress. Do this exercise as part of your normal practice session.

Should I still be exercising during my last month of pregnancy?

If your doctor is in favor of the type of exercise you are doing, by all means continue!

When I am doing the breathing exercises, my extremities begin to shake. What is this reaction?

Your shaking is from too much carbon dioxide to the rest of your body, and is called hyperventilation. Place your cupped hands over your nose and mouth and take slow, deep breaths. This will help you bring the carbon dioxide into proper balance. If you have a paper bag, place the opening over your nose and mouth, and breath slowly.

197

Every time I wash my hair, large hunks come out in my hand. Is this normal?

The increased hormones in your body may indeed cause hair loss. Do not panic. Your hair will feel thinner for a while, but will return to its normal state after pregnancy. Ask your doctor if you should continue taking prenatal vitamins after pregnancy.

Lovemaking has become very difficult since my seventh month. Is there anything we can do to make it more comfortable?

In the latter part of pregnancy, many couples prefer having the man lie behind the woman, because this position does not put pressure on your abdomen. Be flexible about using positions that don't apply much pressure to the abdomen.

I am going to try prepared childbirth, but I'm afraid of being in pain. Do you have any suggestions?

Going to a class for prepared childbirth, and reading books and magazines, will help you prepare. But remember that prolonged or difficult labors that place too much stress on mother and baby should probably be alleviated with some medication.

I've heard about perineal massages, but don't know exactly how or when to do them. What do you recommend?

Perineal massages loosen the tissue around the perineum. Some coaches massage this area for their partners a few weeks prior to delivery. Many midwives do it during delivery, when the head is being delivered. To give a perineal massage, your partner inserts two fingers gently into the vagina and pushes down on the perineum and outward on both sides of the vagina. As your due date gets closer, your partner will be able to insert three fingers to the middle knuckle without your being uncomfortable. However, "uncomfortable" is relative. Some women find perineal massages uncomfortable from the first touch and do *not* want to have them. We think it's a personal choice. Some people say that perineal massages may prevent tearing or the necessity of an episiotomy. We don't know of any definitive studies. However, if you do have your partner give you perineal massages, we recommend them 3 to 5 times a week, starting the thirty-sixth week. And be sure your partner uses a lubricant such as K-Y jelly.

As a coach, I'm concerned I won't be able to handle watching my wife's pain, and I'll ruin a major part of the delivery.

Most coaches have this apprehension but then become so immersed in their duties they forget about it. However, it is important to tell your wife about this concern so you can work it out together. Studies show that the mere *presence* of a coach—you—reduces the discomfort as well as the duration of labor. As a prepared coach, you do have the skills to really help.

We have another child and are concerned about how she will react to her new brother or sister. Do you have any recommendations?

Many hospitals offer sibling classes that are truly wonderful. The children realize that other children are in their situation, and they get to be a part of the pregnancy process. Usually, a nurse runs the program and lets the children hold "newborn" dolls, and diaper and feed them. A film made with young children in mind is usually shown as part of this program. Contact your hospital for further information.

When should I start looking into child care?

We recommend visiting child-care centers, family child-care homes, and in-home caregivers approximately two months before you are due. This will give you an idea of the type of situation you want for your baby, and you will also be able to explore your financial obligations.

How many ultrasounds can be done before affecting the baby? What's the point of one in the last two months of pregnancy?

The U.S. Department of Health states that ultrasounds are safe as long as they are only used as indicated, because they have no long-term data on ultrasounds. During an average pregnancy, an ultrasound is done around 18 to 20 weeks. One will also be performed if you are having an amniocentesis. It will be done prior to the amnio.

If your doctor has any questions at all about the size of your baby or the number of babies, he or she will order an ultrasound.

What is the test called in which you are asked to stimulate your nipples, which makes you have a contraction, and what is the purpose of this test?

This is a stress test, or oxytocin challenge. The purpose is to see how the baby handles the stress of normal labor. You will be asked to stimulate your nipples to spur the production of oxytocin, or you may be given a form of oxytocin until you have three contractions within a ten-minute period. Since contractions tend to cut down the oxygen supply by compressing the placenta, the doctor watches the baby's heart rate to see is there is a change in pattern after the contraction. This test is performed at 34 weeks. The results might dictate induced labor or a cesarean.

What is lightening or dropping?

"Lightening" is another word for the baby's dropping into the pelvis. It is one of the signs that occur two to three weeks before the onset of labor.

My doctor hasn't done an internal exam for a number of months. Shouldn't she be keeping close tabs on the baby?

From your third month until your eighth month, your doctor usually feels your stomach, measures the fetus, checks its position, does an ultrasound, and pushes the fetus in different directions. Unless you are having a problem, your doctor will not do an internal exam during that period of time. However, somewhere between your thirty-sixth and fortieth week, your doctor will do a vaginal exam to see if you are effacing or dilating, and to see if the baby's head has dropped into the pelvic cavity.

Could you please explain the differences between the types of fetal monitors?

The simplest type of fetal monitor is the fetoscope, which looks like a stethoscope and allows the doctor to listen to the baby's heart. Another external monitor uses ultrasound and is strapped around the mother's abdomen; it is the most common monitor in use. An internal fetal monitor is the most accurate of all, and is attached to the scalp of the baby.

How do you know you are in labor?

You have uterine contractions, your bag of waters breaks, and/or you lose your mucus plug. These can happen within a short period of time, or over days.

How will I know if my bag of waters has broken?

You will feel either a gush of fluid running down your leg, or you will notice a little trickle of fluid that you normally wouldn't feel. Please contact your doctor as soon as possible, even if you aren't sure.

Could you recap the first stage of labor for me?

Here's a table for easy reference:

PHASE	CONTRACTION DURATION	CONTRACTION FREQUENCY	LENGTH OF PHASE
Early (0–3 cm)	30 sec.	4–5 min.	7–8 hours
Active (3–7 cm)	60 sec.	3–4 min.	3–5 hours
Trans. (7–10 cm)	70–90 sec.	1 3/4–2 min.	1/2–1 1/2 hours
Pushing	60 sec.	3 min.	1/2 –2+ hours

When should I go to the hospital?

Every doctor has his or her own theory, but pretty standard is the idea that you should get to the hospital when your contractions are 5 minutes apart for 1 hour.

Will they shave my pubic hair in the hospital?

Most hospitals do not require any prep prior to labor unless you are scheduled for a C-section. If you are having a C-section, you will be shaved from the top of your pubic hair to where you cannot see any hair when your legs are closed. Always ask your doctor, so that you are not surprised when you actually do go into labor.

What does a contraction feel like?

Maybe the most-asked question of all time. A contraction feels like a tightening of your muscles from your kidney area in back, then moving around to the front of your belly. You can actually feel your belly become very hard and oddly shaped during a contraction.

Do contractions hurt?

Yes, they feel something like the severe abdominal cramps that you experience during the flu. However, your breathing will help relax you, and make the contractions tolerable.

What is the average heartbeat of a baby during labor?

During labor, a baby's heartbeat varies from 120 to 160 beats per minute. The heartbeat also changes when the mother changes positions, when a contraction is occurring, or when the mother's activity level is changing.

Why do doctors, midwives, and nurses recommend that you walk around during labor?

Research has found that women in an upright position tend to have stronger, more effective contractions. An upright position shortens the first stage of labor by one-third. An upright position takes the pressure off the vena cava, giving both mother and baby a better oxygen supply. This is also why doctors recommend that you don't lie on your back during labor.

What is the reasoning for getting on all-fours during a contraction?

This position takes the weight of the baby off the spine, the pelvic floor, and the rectum.

Should I have a vaginal discharge after the delivery? If so, how long will it last?

Yes, there is a normal bloody discharge after the birth of the baby. It will be heavy and red for the first few days, then it will become pinkish, and finally it will be a light brownish discharge in the last few days. The flow lasts for approximately two weeks. If you notice a heavy bloody discharge or clotting, contact your caregiver immediately.

I heard that you cannot get pregnant if you are nursing. Is this true?

Absolutely not true! You most certainly *can* become pregnant if you are nursing. You may not begin having normal periods until you stop nursing, but you can still ovulate.

Are any support organizations available after I have had a baby?

Yes, your hospital or doctor should be able to provide you with a list of those in your local area.

How long does it take for my uterus to return to its normal size?

About eight weeks.

After I have my baby, can I use tampons instead of sanitary napkins?

Tampons are not recommended because they are uncomfortable when you are healing.

My friend had terrible afterpains for the first couple of days after delivery. Is there anything I can do to avoid this discomfort?

Try to massage your uterus as often as possible to keep the muscles from relaxing, and try to urinate as often as possible even if you don't feel the need. Lie facedown with a pillow under your stomach, putting continuous pressure on your uterus, and try to relax. If none of these methods work, your doctor can prescribe some medication.

I'm concerned whether I'll instantly fall in love with my baby. Is it normal to feel this way?

Of course it is! Real babies are very different from our fantasies of how they're going to look and act. They come out all wrinkled and red, sometimes with a rash, and with hair in places we didn't expect. It takes several days to fall in love with your baby, but it will happen. This is why most hospitals encourage the parents to enjoy the first hour together with your baby, which enhances family bonding.

What exactly does the doctor do during a circumcision?

The boy is usually strapped down or restrained during the procedure. The tip of the penis is usually protected by metal or a plastic bell and the foreskin is then cut off. This is one of the few surgical procedures performed without anesthesia. Over half of all newborn boys are still circumcised in the United States, primarily as a social custom. You make this decision. Not the hospital or the doctor. We recommend that you have your doctor give some type of block to the baby before this procedure is done.

How will I know what my baby wants when it cries?

A baby will cry if it's hungry, needs to suck, has pain from gas/indigestion/colic, is too cold or too hot, has wet diapers or a diaper rash, is constipated, is surprised by sudden loud noises, is overstimulated, wants to be held and touched, or is tired. You'll learn to distinguish—sometimes. Other times you'll never know.

Will I know instinctively how to breastfeed my baby?

As natural and instinctive as breastfeeding may be, there is much that mother and baby have to learn about this basic skill. The natural desire to hold and touch your newborn naturally leads to the act of nursing. If you are unsure, ask your nurse to help the baby onto the breast the first few times. Most maternity nurses are very well versed in the art of breastfeeding, and they have some wonderful "tricks."

How often should I feed my baby?

"On demand" is the usual recommendation. For the first couple of months, this may mean every two hours, and then every four hours, approximately.

I've heard from friends that nipples become very sore and irritated from nursing. What can be done about this?

Most new mothers have sore nipples for the first couple of weeks until the breasts adapt to the strength of the babies' sucking motion. Rub lanolin or Masse cream on your nipples beginning *six weeks* before your due date, and then every time following nursing. Be sure to wash off any cream with warm water before the next feeding. Another option is a nipple shield, a soft plastic device that fits over your nipple. This protects it from actual contact. Consult your physician or LaLeche League if you are having any problems.

What do I do if I start leaking milk in public?

Just take your hands, palm flat, and push hard against your breasts for a few minutes. This pressure will stop the flow of milk.

You can also fold your arms, and press your arms across your breasts. No matter what you do, it will be embarrassing, but at least you won't be leaking all over the place.

I'm planning on returning to work six weeks after the baby is born. How do I prepare the baby for drinking from a bottle?

First, begin using a breast pump as soon as possible after delivery so that *you* are comfortable with the procedure. Then introduce the bottle to your baby a week or two before you return to work. Have someone else give the baby the bottle. If you are returning to work on a full-time basis, prepare three bottles per day; if you are going back part time, prepare two bottles per day.

How will I know if the baby is getting enough to eat?

If the baby appears satisfied at the end of feedings and sleeps for an hour or so and has frequent wet diapers, he's probably getting enough. But if he isn't gaining enough weight, contact your pediatrician.

Am I ready to have my baby?

Yes! And good luck.

Appendix A

Childbirth Educator

Choosing a childbirth educator is very important, because it can "make or break" your attitude toward labor and delivery. Like any other profession, there are good and bad childbirth educators. Most doctors and midwives recommend childbirth classes that are affiliated with their facility. Occasionally, those classes fill up rather quickly, and you will have to locate a childbirth educator on your own. We recommend contacting the 800 number of ASPO/Lamaze for a list of childbirth educators in your particular area. We feel that it is important to speak with the childbirth educator before signing up for class, and ask a few questions beforehand. Remember that the purpose of childbirth classes is to promote a positive response to the childbirth experience, and the childbirth educator plays an important role in preparing expectant parents for childbirth. You will want to know her philosophy and method of teaching (Dick-Read, Lamaze, Bradley, etc.), which will influence her teaching process. Ask when and how often the classes are offered. Some childbirth educators offer one day seminars on Saturdays for working couples, so it pays to ask if they offer that particular service. Ask about the background of the childbirth educator. Is she a certified childbirth educator and by whom is she certified? You will also want to know what information will be covered during the Lamaze program. Most Lamaze instructors try to give the expectant parents information that permits them to make an informed choice, assume a healthier lifestyle, and promote a positive response to the childbirth experience.

Appendix B

Maternal-Child Health Organizations

American College of Nurse-Midwives
1522 K Street NW
Suite 1120
Washington, D.C. 20005
202–289–0171

American College of Obstetricians and Gynecologists
600 Maryland Avenue, SW
Suite 300 East
Washington, D.C. 20024
202–638–5577

American Society for Psychoprophylaxis in Obstetrics
ASPO/Lamaze
1101 Connecticut Avenue NW
Suite 700
Washington, D.C. 20036
202–857–1128

Association for Childbirth at Home, International
P.O. Box 39498
Los Angeles, Cal. 90039
213–667–0839

Association for the Care of Children's Health
3615 Wisconsin Avenue
Washington, D.C. 20016
202–244–1801

Center for the Study of Multiple Births
333 E. Superior, #463–5
Chicago, Ill. 60611
312–266–9093

Cesareans/Support, Education and Concern
22 Forest Road
Framingham, Mass. 01701
617–877–8266

COPE—Coping with the Overall Parenting/Pregnancy Experience
37 Clarendon Street
Boston, Mass. 02116
617–357–5588

Council for Cesarean Awareness
5520 SW 92nd Avenue
Miami, Fla. 33165
305–596–2699

The Fatherhood Project
Families and Work Institute
330 Seventh Avenue
14th Floor
New York, N. Y. 10001
(212) 268-4846

Informal Homebirth/Informed Birth and Parenting
Box 3675
Ann Arbor, Mich. 48106
313–662–6857

International Childbirth Education Association
P.O. Box 20048
Minneapolis, Minn. 55420
612–854–8660

LaLeche League International
9616 Minneapolis Avenue
P.O. Box 1209
Franklin Park, Ill. 60131
312–455–7730

March of Dimes Birth Defects Foundation
1275 Mamaroneck Avenue
White Plains, N.Y. 10605
914–428–7100

National Association of Childbirth Education
3940 Eleventh Street
Riverside, Cal. 92501
714–686–0422

National Association of Parents and Professionals for Safe Alternative
    in Childbirth
P.O. Box 428
Marble Hill, Mo. 63764
314–238–2010

National Center for Education in Maternal and Child Health
38th and R Streets, NW
Washington, D.C. 20057
202–625–8400

National Down's Syndrome Congress
1640 West Roosevelt Road
Chicago, Ill. 60608
312–226–0416

National Institute of Child Health and Human Development
9000 Rockville Pike
Building 31, Room 2A–32
Bethesda, Md. 20205
301–496–4000

National Safety Council
444 North Michigan Avenue
Chicago, Ill. 60611
312–527–4800

Pregnancy Environmental Hotline
  National Birth Defects Center
30 Warren Street
Boston, Mass. 02135
800-322-5014

Society for Nutrition Education
1736 Franklin Street,
Suite 900
Oakland, Cal. 94612
415-444-7133

Parents With Careers Inc.
2513 Oakenshield Drive
Rockville, Md. 20854
800-446-4462, 369-1600 following dial tone

Publications for Parents

American Baby Magazine
249 W. 17th Street
New York, N.Y. 10011

Breastfeeding Abstracts
LaLeche League International, Inc.
9616 Minneapolis Avenue
P.O. Box 1209
Franklin Park, Ill. 60131-8209

Lamaze Parents' Magazine
1840 Wilson Boulevard, Suite 204
Arlington, Va. 22201

Index

Index

hands:
    of newborns, 182
    swelling of, 7, 10
hands and knees position:
    exercises in, 63–64, 97–98, 134
    pushing in, 72
hazardous substances, 128–29
head, of newborns, 138, 181
headaches, 10, 32, 116
Health Maintenance Organizations
        (HMOs), 166
hearing, of newborns, 185
heartburn, 7
heart rate, fetal, 127, 140, 200, 202
hemorrhaging, 75, 117
hemorrhoids, 7
herpes, genital, 140
high blood pressure, 10
hip pain, 32
home:
    change of, 130
    delivery in, 89
    postpartum supplies for, 94–95
    return to, 105–6
hormones, 7–9, 43, 85, 198
    emotions and, 7–8, 87
hospitals, 89
    checking into, 101
    discharge from, 105–6
    fetal monitor use in, 107–8
    internal electrode use in, 109
    IV use in, 107
    maternity floor of, 101–3
    medical procedures in, 107–10
    prepping in, 107
    preregistration at, 89–90
    sibling classes of, 199
    when to go to, 201
household chores, 130, 176–77
human chorionic gonadotropin
        (HCG), 8, 84
hyperventilation, 20–21, 22, 197

ice chips, 42, 80
insomnia, 131
insuranĬe, 26–27, 106, 166–67
    delivery costs and, 89

internal exams, 200
International Childbirth Education
        Association, 148
Isoforane, 117
IVs (intravenous fluids), 107

Kegel exercise, 33, 179, 192

labor:
    descriptions of, 117–20
    false, 38–39, 119
    inducing of, 104, 107, 108,
        112, 120
    packing for, 93
    preterm, 39–40, 119
    prodromal, 40, 112–13
    prolonged, 140, 198
    signs of, 201
    simulated, 156–61
    surprises in, 81
labor, first stage of (dilation),
        35–38, 40–44, 101–4, 201
    active phase of, 36, 41–43, 114,
        116, 158–59, 201
    bloody show in, 37, 118
    breaking of bag of waters in,
        36–37, 41, 117, 118, 146,
        148, 201
    checking in during, 101
    dilation in, 37–38, 42, 43
    drugs administered in, 112, 116
    early phase of, 36, 40–41, 119,
        157–58, 201
    effacement in, 38
    maternity floor and, 101–3
    nurse procedures in, 103–4
    simulated, 157–60
    transition phase of, 36, 43–44,
        118, 159–60, 201
    see also contractions
labor, second stage of (pushing and
        birth), 68–74
    birth in, 73–74
    breathing in, 77–79
    drugs administered in, 112, 115,
        116, 117

218

Index

About the Authors

O. Robin Sweet was a nurse for over ten years, and owned and operated a nanny placement agency for six years. She has been a certified Lamaze instructor for twenty years, and focuses her classes on the special needs of pregnant working women. The author of a previous book, entitled *The Nanny Connection,* she lives in Piedmont, California.

Patty Bryan, coauthor of *Sharing the Caring,* is a freelance writer and editor.